Battling Aflatoxins - Advances in Food and Feed Research

Edited by Jean-Claude Assaf

Published in London, United Kingdom

Battling Aflatoxins - Advances in Food and Feed Research
http://dx.doi.org/10.5772/intechopen.1005711
Edited by Jean-Claude Assaf

Contributors
Andréia Bianchini, Donna M. Morrison, Ghosoon Albahri, Heba Hellany, Jean-Claude Assaf, Marianela Bossa, María Laura Chiotta, María Silvina Alaniz-Zanon, Nethra Puttaswamy, Ram K. Shrestha, Rayan Kashmar, Sofía Noemí Chulze

First published in London, United Kingdom, 2025 by IntechOpen
IntechOpen is the global imprint of INTECHOPEN LIMITED, registered in England and Wales, registration number: 11086078, 167-169 Great Portland Street, London, W1W 5PF, United Kingdom

For EU product safety concerns: IN TECH d.o.o., Prolaz Marije Krucifikse Kozulić 3, 51000 Rijeka, Croatia, info@intechopen.com or visit our website at intechopen.com.

British Library Cataloguing-in-Publication Data
A catalogue record for this book is available from the British Library

Battling Aflatoxins - Advances in Food and Feed Research
Edited by Jean-Claude Assaf
p. cm.
Print ISBN 978-1-83634-452-0
Online ISBN 978-1-83634-451-3
eBook (PDF) ISBN 978-1-83634-453-7

Meet the editor

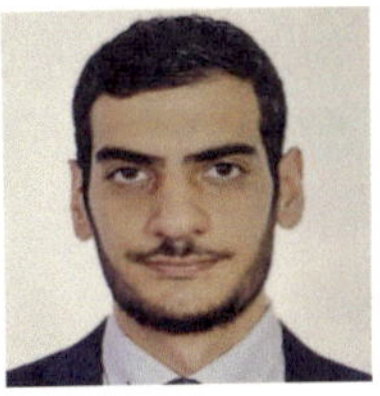

Dr. Jean-Claude Assaf is an Associate Professor of Chemical Engineering at the University of Balamand (UOB), holding a Ph.D. in chemistry and microbiology. He has received national and international awards, including LIRA and the French Society of Microbiology Prize. His expertise spans mycotoxicology, chemical process design, simulation, and food science. Dr. Assaf owns multiple patents, has authored peer-reviewed publications, and is a frequent speaker at scientific conferences. He serves as Chair of the International Chemical Engineering Advisory Board and advisor of the Society of Petroleum Engineers (SPE) Student Chapter. He has edited several books and guest-edited journals such as Processes and Applied Chemical Engineering, actively collaborating with academia and industry on multidisciplinary research.

Contents

Preface

Aflatoxins continue to represent a persistent challenge in the global food and feed industry, threatening both human health and food security. These toxic secondary metabolites, primarily produced by *Aspergillus flavus* and *Aspergillus parasiticus*, contaminate a wide range of crops, including maize, peanuts, and tree nuts, particularly under tropical and subtropical conditions. Their impact spans from acute toxicity and carcinogenicity in humans and animals to economic losses due to strict international regulatory limits and reduced trade opportunities.

The battle against aflatoxins is multidimensional. It involves early detection, prevention, effective post-harvest control, and informed policy implementation. Scientific progress in fields such as biotechnology, microbiology, analytical chemistry, food engineering, and agricultural management has yielded promising methods for monitoring and reducing aflatoxin levels in food systems. However, integrating these innovations into scalable and sustainable strategies remains a formidable task.

This book, *Battling Aflatoxins – Advances in Food and Feed Research*, brings together recent research and applied insights from leading scholars and professionals worldwide. The contributions in this volume span a wide range of topics, including aflatoxin detection, biocontrol strategies using non-aflatoxigenic strains and advances in food processing techniques to reduce contamination. Notably, the book offers both foundational scientific knowledge and practical approaches that can be adapted to various agricultural contexts. The interdisciplinary nature of this work reflects the complexity of aflatoxin contamination and the need for collaborative, cross-sectoral efforts. The book is designed to support researchers, food safety authorities, agricultural extension services, and policymakers in their efforts to mitigate the impact of mycotoxins on human health, animal welfare, and global food systems.

I want to express my sincere gratitude to all contributing authors for their dedication, scientific rigor, and valuable insights. Special thanks go to IntechOpen for providing a platform that bridges science and society by making cutting-edge research freely accessible to the global community. I also acknowledge the support of my institution, the University of Balamand (UOB) for encouraging applied research and innovation in food safety and public health.

I hope this book will serve as a catalyst for further research, informed decision-making, and international cooperation aimed at eliminating the threats posed by aflatoxins and ensuring a safer and more resilient food supply for future generations.

Jean-Claude Assaf
Faculty of Engineering (FOE),
Chemical Engineering Department,
University of Balamand (UOB),
Koura, Lebanon

Chapter 1

Introductory Chapter: Confronting the Global Challenge of Aflatoxins in Food and Feed Systems

Jean-Claude Assaf

1. Introduction

Aflatoxins represent one of the most insidious and persistent threats to food and feed safety worldwide. These naturally occurring mycotoxins are produced primarily by *Aspergillus flavus* and *Aspergillus parasiticus* fungi, which proliferate under hot and humid conditions that favor fungal growth and toxin biosynthesis. Found predominantly in staple crops such as maize, peanuts, tree nuts, and cereals, aflatoxins contaminate agricultural commodities both pre- and post-harvest, posing a significant challenge to food security, animal health, trade, and public safety [1, 2].

The global distribution of aflatoxins is intrinsically linked to climatic factors and agricultural practices. Developing countries, particularly those in tropical and subtropical regions, bear the brunt of aflatoxin contamination due to inadequate storage infrastructures, limited regulatory oversight, and the prevalence of smallholder farming [3]. However, climate change and increasing temperatures have begun to shift the geographical boundaries of aflatoxin prevalence, making it a growing concern even in temperate regions. Aflatoxins are notorious for their toxicological potency. Among the different types, aflatoxin B1 is the most carcinogenic and is classified by the International Agency for Research on Cancer [4] as a Group 1 human carcinogen. Chronic exposure to aflatoxins is associated with hepatocellular carcinoma, stunted growth in children, immune suppression, and increased vulnerability to infectious diseases [5]. In animals, aflatoxin-contaminated feed leads to reduced productivity, organ damage, and mortality, particularly in poultry, cattle, and swine.

Despite decades of research and the availability of several mitigation strategies, aflatoxin management remains a multifaceted problem. The resilience of the *Aspergillus* species, combined with poor post-harvest handling, inconsistent policy implementation, and insufficient awareness, contributes to the persistence of the problem. Furthermore, the economic impact of aflatoxin contamination extends beyond public health. It affects trade balances by limiting export opportunities for contaminated commodities, especially in regions where regulatory limits are strictly enforced [6].

IntechOpen

2. The complexity of aflatoxin contamination

Aflatoxin contamination is influenced by a multitude of factors, ranging from environmental to socio-economic. Biologically, the interaction between host plant susceptibility and fungal aggressiveness plays a pivotal role. Abiotic stressors such as drought, heat, and insect damage further exacerbate fungal colonization and toxin accumulation [7]. This complexity necessitates a comprehensive, interdisciplinary approach to aflatoxin control. Monitoring and detection are key components of aflatoxin risk management. Recent advances in rapid diagnostic tools, including immunoassays and molecular techniques, have improved the ability to detect aflatoxins at low concentrations. However, the accessibility of these tools in resource-limited settings remains a concern. Analytical laboratories capable of enforcing regulatory thresholds are often concentrated in urban centers, leaving rural areas underserved [3].

3. Integrated strategies for mitigation

Effective control of aflatoxins involves integrated management strategies that span the entire value chain. These include:

- *Pre-harvest interventions*, such as the development of resistant crop varieties, biological control using atoxigenic strains of *Aspergillus*, and improved agronomic practices like crop rotation and irrigation management [7].

- *Post-harvest techniques*, including proper drying, use of hermetic storage technologies, and chemical treatments to inhibit fungal growth [6].

- *Policy and regulation*, which necessitate stringent enforcement of aflatoxin limits in food and feed, along with surveillance systems and consumer education programs [1].

Biological control, particularly through competitive exclusion with non-aflatoxigenic strains, has shown promising results in several countries. These biocontrol products can significantly reduce aflatoxin levels in treated fields. Moreover, community-based approaches that combine technological, behavioral, and institutional innovations are crucial to sustaining progress [7].

4. Research and future directions

Innovative research is expanding the frontiers of aflatoxin management. Advances in genomics and transcriptomics are enabling a better understanding of the regulatory mechanisms controlling aflatoxin biosynthesis.

Nanotechnology is being explored for improved detection and detoxification methods. Additionally, predictive modeling is aiding in forecasting contamination risks based on weather data, allowing for timely interventions [2]. A growing area of interest is the exploration of sustainable and nature-based solutions for aflatoxin prevention. This includes the incorporation of biopesticides derived from natural antagonists, as well as the use of plant-based extracts that inhibit fungal growth or

DOI: http://dx.doi.org/10.5772/intechopen.1011379

neutralize aflatoxins. There is also considerable potential in combining traditional knowledge with modern scientific methods to develop culturally appropriate and scalable interventions. Furthermore, aflatoxin mitigation is increasingly being recognized within the broader framework of the Sustainable Development Goals (SDGs), particularly in relation to food security, health, and economic growth [3]. By aligning aflatoxin control strategies with sustainability agendas, stakeholders can create long-lasting impacts that go beyond contamination reduction.

Nonetheless, the fight against aflatoxins is far from over. Global collaboration, equitable technology transfer, and sustained investments in research and capacity building are imperative. There is also a need for harmonized international standards and inclusive policies that consider the realities of smallholder farmers and vulnerable populations.

5. Conclusion

Aflatoxins remain a global concern with profound implications for public health, agriculture, and trade. The battle against these contaminants requires a coordinated, science-driven response that bridges research, policy, and practice. As our understanding deepens and technologies evolve, the prospects for effective control improve. The pursuit of safe food and feed systems must continue, rooted in innovation, collaboration, and an unwavering commitment to health and sustainability.

Author details

Jean-Claude Assaf
Microbial Engineering Laboratory, Faculty of Engineering, Department of Chemical Engineering, University of Balamand, Tripoli, Lebanon

*Address all correspondence to: jeanclaude.assaf@balamand.edu.lb

References

[1] Williams JH, Phillips TD, Jolly PE, Stiles JK, Jolly CM, Aggarwal D. Human aflatoxicosis in developing countries: A review of toxicology, exposure, potential health consequences, and interventions. The American Journal of Clinical Nutrition. 2004;**80**(5):1106-1122

[2] Milani J. Ecological conditions affecting mycotoxin production in cereals: A review. Veterinární Medicína. 2013;**58**(8):405-411

[3] Wild CP, Gong YY. Mycotoxins and human disease: A largely ignored global health issue. Carcinogenesis. 2010;**31**(1):71-82

[4] IARC. Monographs on the Evaluation of Carcinogenic Risks to Humans. Vol. 100F. Lyon, France: World Health Organization; 2012

[5] Turner PC, Burley VJ, Rothwell JA, White KLM, Cade JE, Wild CP, et al. Dietary wheat reduction decreases the level of urinary deoxynivalenol in UK adults. Journal of Exposure Science & Environmental Epidemiology [Internet]. Jul 2008;**18**(5):392-399. DOI: 10.1038/sj.jes.7500611 [cited 2025 Jul 2]

[6] Hell K, Mutegi C. Aflatoxin control and prevention strategies in key crops of sub-Saharan Africa. African Journal of Microbiology Research. 2011;**5**(5):459-466

[7] Bandyopadhyay R, Ortega-Beltran A, Akande A, Mutegi C, Atehnkeng J, Kaptoge L, et al. Biological control of aflatoxins in Africa: Current status and potential challenges in the face of climate change. World Mycotoxin Journal. 2016;**9**(5):771-789

Chapter 2

Unveiling the Hidden Threat of Aflatoxins: Occurrence, Biochemical Pathways, Regulatory Standards, and Health Risks

Heba Hellany, Rayan Kashmar, Ghosoon Albahri and Jean-Claude Assaf

Abstract

Aflatoxins, toxic secondary metabolites produced by *Aspergillus* genus, represent a significant risk to food safety and public health. They are known for their hepatotoxic and carcinogenic affects, which pose severe health risks to human and animals. This chapter delves into the biochemistry of aflatoxins, exploring their diversity and the structural characteristics of the four major aflatoxins (B1, B2, G1, and G2). Furthermore, it explores the complex biosynthesis pathway for aflatoxin B1 (AFB1) in *Aspergillus* genus involving 27 steps that are mainly regulated by specific gene clusters and transcription factors (*aflR* and *aflJ*), alongside environmental modulators such as carbon and nitrogen. This chapter also addresses the contamination of various crops by aflatoxins, driven by many environmental factors such as temperature, moisture, and pH leading to considerable economic losses and strict regulatory limits set by the European Union (EU) and the U.S. Food and Drug Administration (FDA). Finally, the health risks associated with aflatoxin exposure, particularly hepatotoxicity, hepatocellular carcinoma, mitochondrial damage, and apoptosis, with insights into molecular pathways are reported in this chapter.

Keywords: aflatoxins, biosynthesis, hepatotoxicity, carcinogenesis, detoxification, pathways

1. Introduction

Mycotoxins, secondary metabolites produced by filamentous fungi, have garnered considerable attention due to their diverse impacts on human and animal health. The term "mycotoxin" was first introduced in the UK during the 1960s to describe a toxin identified in peanuts used as animal feed [1]. This toxin was associated with the sudden deaths of turkeys following the consumption of contaminated peanuts, a phenomenon known as Turkey-X disease [1]. Aflatoxins are a class of mycotoxins produced through the secondary metabolism of filamentous fungi belonging to the genus *Aspergillus*, specifically within the section *Flavi*. The main toxigenic species responsible for aflatoxin production are *A. flavus* and *A. parasiticus* [2]. The International Agency for Research on Cancer (IARC) has classified aflatoxins (including AFB1, AFB2, AFG1, and AFG2) as Group 1 carcinogens, with AFB1 being the most potent hepatotoxic compound and a significant hepatic carcinogen [1–3]. AFB1 undergoes biotransformation in the liver, where cytochrome P450 (CYP 450) enzymes, mainly CYP1A2 and CYP3A4, metabolize it into various DNA adducts. These DNA adducts contribute to its mutagenic and carcinogenic effects, particularly hepatocellular carcinoma (HCC) [4]. Globally, it is estimated that 4.5 billion people are exposed to AFB1, with 5-28% of global HCC cases attributed to aflatoxins exposure [2, 3]. Co-exposure to AFB1 and hepatitis B virus (HBV) amplifies the risk of HCC development by up to 30-fold, causing a severe health challenge in developing countries where both factors are prevalent. Similarly, a relationship exists between AFB1 exposure and hepatitis C virus (HCV), further elevating HCC risk [2]. In addition to their hepatotoxic and carcinogenic effects, aflatoxins can cause acute toxicity, where high-dose intake over a short period leads to severe aflatoxicosis outbreaks, often resulting in fatalities due to liver damage and systemic poisoning [5]. Chronic exposure to low doses over extended periods leads to immune suppression, growth stunting, and an increased risk of liver cancer, including structural liver damage such as congestion, swelling, necrosis, and discoloration [5]. Additionally, aflatoxin intake generates oxidative stress, exacerbating liver damage and contributing to both acute and chronic cellular injuries [6].

AFB1 poses significant challenges due to its low molecular weight, chemical stability, and resistance to thermal processes such as autoclaving, boiling, cooking, and fermentation, which further complicates its elimination from contaminated food sources [2]. The contamination of natural products and their by-products occur in two distinct phases: The first involves the infection of developing crops, while the second includes contamination at any stage from maturation to consumption. This highlights the importance of implementing both pre- and post-harvest management strategies to minimize aflatoxin contamination effectively [3]. Furthermore, certain nutrients in grains play a role in the risk of aflatoxin production; for example, lipids in ground substrates significantly increase this risk, while sugars and proteins also contribute to the production of aflatoxins [3].

This chapter explores the biochemistry of aflatoxins, focusing on their structural diversity, biosynthesis in *Aspergillus* species, and regulatory mechanisms involving gene clusters and environmental factors. It examines the contamination of crops driven by environmental conditions and regulatory limits set by the EU and FDA. Additionally, it highlights the health risks associated with aflatoxin exposure, including hepatotoxicity, hepatocellular carcinoma, and cellular damage, with insights into the underlying molecular pathways.

2. Biochemistry of aflatoxins

The most toxic mycotoxins are aflatoxins, which are mostly produced by *Aspergillus* species. They can cause both acute and chronic toxicities, with the severe and recognized ones being immunotoxicity, mutagenicity, and genotoxicity [7]. Despite being a global issue, developing nations in tropical and sub-tropical regions are more affected by aflatoxins in terms of their negative effects on social life, the economy, and health. The region's highest incidence of hepatocellular carcinoma and acute aflatoxicosis outbreak episodes have historically been linked to agricultural products from SSA countries, such as Gambia, Uganda, Kenya, and Tanzania, and SEA countries, such as China, Thailand, Vietnam, and Indonesia [8]. Over 18 distinct types of aflatoxin can arise naturally or as a result of carryover in foods and feeds. Toxigenic molds naturally produce around 13 different types of aflatoxins, some of which can be metabolized by humans, animals, or other microorganisms to produce derivatives that are still toxic but typically less potent than the parent molecules. The economy and public health are most concerned about AFB1, AFB2, AFG1, and AFG2 because of their high prevalence and high toxicities. Aflatoxin M1 (AFM1), on the other hand, poses a particular risk to the safety of dairy products due to its high toxicity and potential for human cancer, as well as the fact that it is typically passed on in the milk of nursing animals fed aflatoxin B1-contaminated feed [9].

2.1 Molecular weight and structure

Aflatoxin structurally consists of a coumarin nucleus to which a difuran moiety is attached on one side and either a pentone ring or a six-membered lactone ring is attached on the other. Aflatoxin is a difuranocournarin or difurocoumarin that is synthesized through the polyketide pathway. Accordingly, aflatoxins can be divided into two major categories: difurocoumarolactones with the aflatoxin G series as the primary representatives, usually comprising AFG1, AFG2, AFGM1, AFGM2, and AFG2a; and difurocoumarocyclopentenones, which are generally composed of aflatoxin B series and derivatives, as presented in **Table 1**. Even though AFB3 (also known as aflatoxin B3) does not have the distinctive six-membered lactone ring, it is typically regarded as belonging to the latter group [11]. Aflatoxin B1 and G1 have the molecular formulas $C_{17}H1_2O6$ and $C_{17}H_{12}O_7$, respectively; aflatoxins B2 and G2 were discovered to be the dihydro-compounds of the $C_{17}H_{14}O_6$ and $C_{17}H_{14}O_7$ parent compounds [10].

2.2 Properties of aflatoxins

It is commonly known that aflatoxins are toxic to both humans and animals when consumed through food and feed, and that they are linked to both acute and chronic illnesses [12]. However, the type of aflatoxin and the host are the primary determinants of the level of toxicity and toxicological effects. AFM1 is just as toxic as AFG1, but AFB1 is by far the most toxic aflatoxin, followed by AFG1, AFB2, and AFG2 [13]. Public health is still concerned about the other less toxic aflatoxins and those deemed "non-toxic" or detoxified because of their intrinsic, albeit weak, toxicities, with potencies ranging from 0.1 to 50% in comparison with AFB1 [14]. Notably, aflatoxins with hydrated (AFB2a, AFG2a, AFM2a, AFQ2a, AFG2a, and AFGM2a) or saturated (AFG2, AFGM2, and AFM2) terminal furan rings are the least toxic, suggesting that the C8 = C9 double bond of this furan moiety is essential to aflatoxins' toxicity [15]. The most toxic of these substances is AFB1, and its metabolites exhibit a range of biological activities, such as acute toxicity, teratogenicity, mutagenicity, and carcinogenicity [16]. Thus, it has been well-documented that these compounds cause HCC in both humans and animals. Apart from DNA adduction, AFB1-induced oxidative stress and inflammation can also contribute to the development of cancer [6]. Chronic exposure to aflatoxins impairs immunity and disrupts the metabolism

Aflatoxin	Molecular formula	Molecular weight	Structure	Melting point	$[\alpha]D^{23}$
B_1	$C_{17}H_{12}O_6$	312	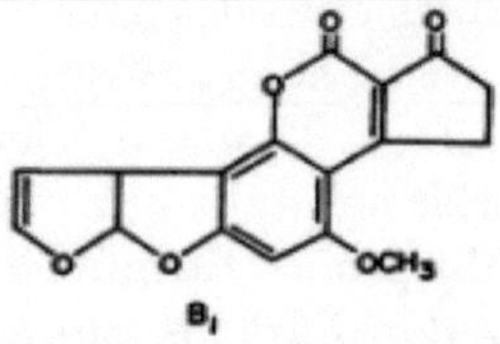	268-269*	−559
B_2	$C_{17}H_{14}O_6$	314	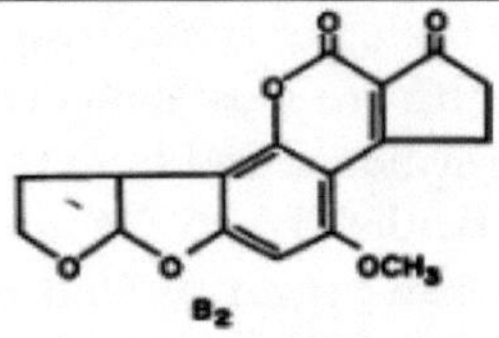	286-289*	−492
G_1	$C_{17}H_{12}O_7$	328	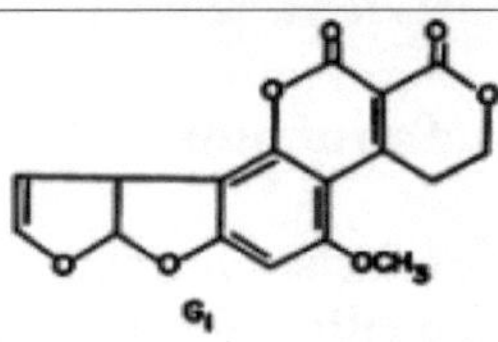	244-246*	−533
G_2	$C_{17}H_{14}O_7$	330	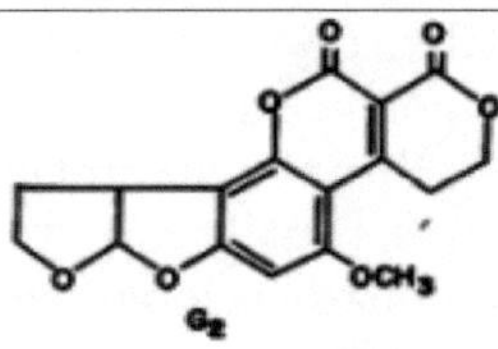	237-240*	−473

Decomposes.

Table 1.
Structure and molecular weights of the four major aflatoxins (B1, B2, G1, and G2) [10].

of proteins and several other vital micronutrients in farm and lab animals. Over 40% of the burden of disease in the developing nations with short lifespans is caused by health factors, including HIV infection, which is adversely affected by aflatoxin exposure and the toxic effects of aflatoxins on immunity and nutrition [17]. Although developed-country methods of managing aflatoxins are impractical in developing-country contexts due to food systems and economics, the use of food additives to shield farm animals from the toxin may also offer novel, cost-effective ways to safeguard human populations [17].

3. Aflatoxin biosynthesis in *Aspergillus* genus

Only a limited number of fungi are able to produce aflatoxins, but two species, *A. flavus* and *A. parasiticus*, are the most common species responsible for their production and they are significant colonizers of agricultural crops [18].

3.1 The aflatoxin biosynthetic gene cluster

In the genus *Aspergillus*, DNA is organized on eight chromosomes, and genes responsible for aflatoxin synthesis are all located in cluster 54. This cluster resides 80 kb from the telomere on the third chromosome [19]. DNA analysis showed

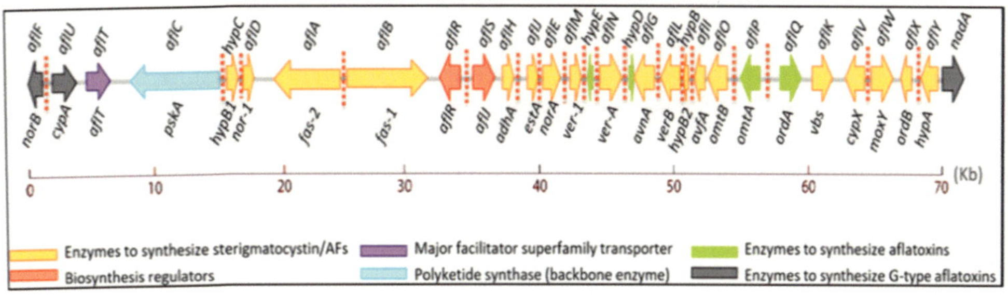

Figure 1.
Structure of aflatoxin biosynthesis gene cluster in Aspergillus species [21].

that both strains of *A. flavus* and *A. parasiticus* share about 96% similarity in this gene cluster [20]. Research on the aflatoxin gene cluster is comprehensive in both *A. flavus* and *A. parasiticus*, revealing that the genes within the cluster share a high degree of similarity, with homology ranging from 90 to 99 % between these two fungal species [19]. Comprising 30 genes, the activation of this cluster is predominantly controlled by two regulatory genes, *aflR* and *aflS*, as shown in **Figure 1** [19].

3.2 Aflatoxin biosynthesis pathway

The biosynthesis of aflatoxin in *Aspergillus* is a long and complicated process that requires about 27 enzyme-catalyzed steps involving at least 15 steps as intermediates [22]. The main substrates that contribute to aflatoxins biosynthesis are 1-Acetyl-CoA and 9-Malonyl-coA [6]. Cytochromes P-450 enzymes are important for aflatoxin production, as they help attach functional groups such as methyl and acetyl groups during the biosynthesis process. Four stable metabolites are produced during the AFB1: norsoloric acid, versicolorin A, sterigmatocystin, and aflatoxin B1 [19].

3.2.1 Synthesis of norsoloric acid (NOR)

The first step of the AFs biosynthetic pathway is the production of norsoloric acid (NOR). NOR is a red-orange metabolite in certain mutant strains and a crucial step in the aflatoxin biosynthetic pathway. This process begins with the formation of hexanoate units (from acetyl-CoA and malonyl-CoA) that then undergo chain elongation and structural transformations into the first stable metabolite, NOR [19, 21]. The genes involved include:

aflA (fatty acid synthase α) and *aflB* (fatty acid synthase β): Encode fatty acid synthase subunits α and β. They are essential for the production of NorS, which is critical for the formation of the hexanoyl primer. The primer then combines with malonyl-CoA to create norsolorinic acid anthrone (NAA), thus, facilitating the conversion of hexanoate units into a polyketide structure [19, 21].

aflC: Codes for polyketide synthase, which elongates the polyketide chain, ultimately forming NAA. The primer then combines with malonyl-CoA to create norsolorinic acid anthrone (NAA) [19, 21].

hypC: Encodes an enzyme (NAA oxidase) that catalyzes the conversion of NAA into NOR [19, 21].

3.2.2 Conversion of NOR into versicolorin a (VERA)

This conversion involves multiple steps. Firstly, NOR is converted into averantin (AVN) through a step involving the *aflD* gene. *aflD* encodes a ketoreductase that modifies norsolorinic acid into AVN by converting a keto group into a hydroxyl group. Then, the conversion of AVN into 5′-Hydroxyaverantin (HAVN) where *aflG* encodes a cytochrome P-450 monooxygenase that hydroxylates AVN into 5′-hydroxyaverantin (HAVN), and *aflH* (adhA) encodes an alcohol dehydrogenase converting HAVN to 5′-oxoaverantin (OAVN). *aflK*, an OAVN cyclase, then catalyzes the transformation of OAVN into averufin (AVF) [19, 21, 23]. Subsequent reactions involve additional genes (*aflI, aflV, aflW, aflJ aflK, aflL*). In the final step to versicolorin A (VERA), *aflL*, a cytochrome P-450 monooxygenase/desaturase, converts the tetrahydrofuran ring into a dihydrobisfuran ring, marking the last transformation step toward B or G-type aflatoxins [19, 21, 23].

3.2.3 Conversion of VERA into sterigmatocystin

In the first step, VERA is converted into demethylsterigmatocystin (DMST), and the gene *aflM* is involved in this conversion, which encodes a ketoreductase. In addition, four other genes (*aflN, aflY, aflX, and aflO*) contribute to the conversion of DMST into sterigmatocystin (ST), which is the precursor to AFB1 in other species [19, 21].

3.2.4 Conversion into AFB1

The *aflP* gene in *A. parasiticus* encodes an O-methyltransferase critical for converting sterigmatocystin (ST) into O-methylsterigmatocystin (OMST). The final step of the long pathway includes the conversion of OMST into AFB1 and it involves different genes: *aflQ, hypB, aflE*, and *hype* [19, 21]. Notably, the final step in aflatoxin production involves the hype gene and requires an NADPH-dependent monooxygenase, *ordA* [19, 24].

3.3 Molecular regulation of aflatoxin biosynthesis

3.3.1 Regulators specific to the aflatoxin cluster

- *aflR*: Among the genes identified as involved in aflatoxin synthesis, only the gene *aflR* acts as a transcription factor [24]. The aflatoxin biosynthetic pathway is mainly regulated by *aflR* gene. In *A. flavus*, it can binds to at least 17 genes within the cluster, triggering the activation of the aflatoxin synthesis pathway [19]. Thus, it is a transcription factor that contains 444 amino acids and include different domains regulating the aflatoxin biosynthesis. In addition, it is considered a zinc cluster transcription factor because it contains the $Cys_6\_Zn_2$ domain, which is crucial for DNA binding, and it is homologous to Gal4-type family of transcription factors, which are specific to the fungal kingdom [24]. Another domain is the nuclear localization signal domain, which is rich in arginine residues shows 71% similarity between *A. flavus* and *A. parasiticus* [24]. This domain is required for the movement of *aflR* from the cytoplasm to the nucleus [21]. *AflR* binds specifically to the palindromic sequence 5′-TCG(N5)CGA-3′ [19, 21, 24]. *AflR* is considered as an activator of the aflatoxin gene cluster. In *A. flavus*, increased expression of *aflR* leads to the upregulation of multiple aflatoxin genes, resulting in a 50-fold increase in aflatoxin production [19]. *AflR* retains the palindromic sequence in its own promoter, suggesting that, in addition to regulating the AF gene cluster, *aflR* may also regulate its own expression [19, 21]. In a study conducted by Price et al. [25], it was observed that *aflR*-mutated strains of *A. parasiticus* are unable to synthesize aflatoxins due to the absence of most AF genes in the cluster.

- *aflS*: The *aflS* gene (previously named *aflJ*) is essential for aflatoxin production in *A. parasiticus*. *aflS*, encoding a 438-amino acid protein, lacks significant homology with other known proteins and is located next to *aflR* in the aflatoxin biosynthetic cluster [19, 24]. *aflR* regulates *aflS*, and the two genes share a 737-bp intergenic region [19, 21, 24]. The disruption of *aflS* in *A. parasiticus* led to a 5- to 20-fold reduction in certain AFB1 genes (e.g., *aflC, aflD, aflM,* and *aflP*) and a consequent loss in AF intermediate synthesis [19]. Although the precise mechanism by which aflS enhances transcription of AF pathway genes is unclear, it is suggested that *aflR* and *aflS* may form a protein complex that binds specific promoter sites, especially those for early-stage genes such as *aflC* and *aflD*, to increase AFB1 synthesis [19]. Other studies in *A. flavus* and *A. parasiticus* revealed that *aflS* interacts with *aflR* (but not directly with biosynthetic enzymes), suggesting a co-regulatory function; however, additional research is needed to confirm this hypothesis [19, 21]. Thus, the three possible roles of *aflS* are as follows [21]:

- It may act as a coactivator for *aflR*, though deleting *aflS* has minimal impact on *aflR* transcript levels.

- *AflS* may significantly influence the early genes involved in aflatoxin production.

- *AflS* may be a regulatory factor that enhances or supports the transcription of other genes in the aflatoxin biosynthesis pathway, specifically *aflC, aflD, aflM,* and *aflP* [21].

3.3.2 Other transcription regulators

- Velvet complex: The velvet complex is comprised of *VeA, LaeA,* and *VelB,* and it is a light-sensitive complex. Thus, it is a conserved regulatory unit in filamentous fungi that controls the secondary metabolite production and fungal development [5, 21]. While *VelC* shows limited roles in the development or toxin production in *A. flavus*, the Velvet complex has been identified across multiple fungal species, including *Aspergillus* [5]. In *A. flavus*, *veA* and *laeA* are crucial for aflatoxin production and normal development, influencing both sclerotia formation and conidiation. The suppression of these genes reduces quorum sensing and pathogenicity on seeds, with mutants producing less conidia and aflatoxins and showing impaired intracellular invasion and lipid degradation [5].

In *A. flavus,* the mutation of *veA* blocks aflatoxin formation. Similarly, in *A. parasiticus*, laeA mutants show no detectable expression of *aflR* or other AF biosynthesis genes. Conversely, overexpression of *laeA* in *A. parasiticus* leads to increased *aflR* expression and enhanced AF production [23].

- G proteins: G-protein pathways are general transcription regulators, serving as signaling transducers in response to external stimuli. G proteins consist of three subunits: α, β, and γ. In aflatoxin biosynthesis, it has been shown that two Gα subunits (GanB and FadA) inhibit ST/AF biosynthesis by suppressing *aflR* activity; however, the Gβ and Gγ subunits (SfaD and GpgA) promote St and AF synthesis, suggesting the ole of G protein subunits in ST/AF biosynthesis [21, 23].

- Response to oxidative stress:

- The response to oxidative stress and the secondary metabolism are closely interconnected in many filamentous fungi including *A. flavus* and *A. parasiticus* [5, 21]. Secondary metabolism is often activated by cellular oxidative stress, with different proteins, with many proteins, specifically bZIP transcription factors such as *AtfB, AtfA, ApYapA, NapA,* and *AP-1* that regulate these processes [5]. For instance, in *A. parasiticus*, the expression of *AtfB* aligns with aflatoxin production. In addition, *AtfB* associates with *AP-1* to increase the expression of aflatoxin biosynthetic genes [5]. Other proteins like *MsnA* influences both oxidative stress and secondary metabolism. For example, the deletion of *MsnA* in *A. flavus* and *A. parasiticus* species increases the aflatoxin production and the reactive oxygen species production [5].

- Global transcription factors in fungi:

- The *aflR-aflJ* intergenic region in toxigenic *Aspergillus* species contains binding sites for environmental-responsive transcription factors [5]. *CreA, AreA,* and *PacC* are global transcription regulators that respond to environmental stimuli play roles in metabolic regulation of aflatoxins biosynthesis. *CreA*, a zinc-finger transcription factor, is activated by carbon sources and controls metabolic activities accordingly. Similarly, *AreA* regulates nitrogen metabolism and includes a binding site in the *aflS-aflR* intergenic region that may enhance aflatoxin production [21, 26]. Both *CreA* and *AreA,* along with *PacC,* a regulator sensitive to pH changes, are global transcription factors involved in signaling cascades, including those involving cAMP-dependent protein kinase A, to activate the aflatoxin gene cluster [21, 26].

4. Contamination of food products with *Aspergillus* species and aflatoxins

4.1 Common contaminated food products worldwide

Aflatoxins, a type of mycotoxins, are toxic secondary metabolites produced by certain *Aspergillus* species and pose a significant threat to food safety worldwide [27, 28]. Around 25% of the world's food crops and their products are contaminated each year, leading to significant agricultural and industrial losses [29, 30]. Their occurrence has been reported in a wide variety of food products, including nuts, grains, spices, milk, and dairy products, due to contamination at various stages of production, processing, and storage [31]. **Table 2** summarizes the occurrence and levels of aflatoxins in diverse food products from different countries, highlighting the global nature of this

Country	Food product	Number of samples	Aflatoxin Types	Mean	References
India	Chilgoza pine nuts	58	Total AFs	0.493913 ± 0.088785 μg/kg	[32]
Pakistan	Pistachios with shell	15	Total AFs/AFB1	Total AFs: 4.90 ± 0.90 μg/kg AFB1: 4.20 ± 0.75 μg/kg	[33]
	Pistachios without shell	16		Total AFs: 7.10 ± 0.85 μg/kg AFB1: 5.80 ± 0.60 μg/kg	
	Peanuts with shell	14		Total AFs: 6.10 ± 1.30 μg/kg AFB1: 5.50 ± 1.30 μg/kg	
	Peanuts without shell	11		Total AFs: 7.30 ± 1.80 μg/kg AFB1: 5.90 ± 1.10 μg/kg	
Nigeria	Raw groundnuts	15	Total AFs	0.029–0.03378 μg/kg	[34]
	Roasted cashew nuts	27		0.0001–0.0068 μg/kg	
Democratic Republic of Congo	Maize	30	Total AFs/AFB1	Total AFs: 3.03-165.2 μg/kg AFB1: 1.5-81.67 μg/kg	[35]
Uganda	Maize	240	Total AFs	Mid-altitude moist zone: 20.54 μg/kg	[36]
				Mid-altitude dry zone: 18.02 μg/kg	
				Highland: 12.35 μg/kg	
Nyanza, Kenya	Maize	71	Total AFs	7-65 μg/kg	[37]
Turkey	Raw milk	48	AFM1	0.03663-0.10437 μg/L	[38]
Ethiopia	Raw milk	100	AFM1	0.39-0.69 μg/L	[39]
Lebanon	Raw milk	701	AFM1	0.035 ± 0.051 μg/L	[40]
	Pasteurized and UHT milk	11		0.069 ± 0.068 μg/L	

Country	Food product	Number of samples	Aflatoxin Types	Mean	References
Ireland	Spices: Pepper	130	Total AFs	0.45 μg/kg	[41]
	Chili			3.23 μg/kg	
	Curry			0.40 μg/kg	
	Cayenne			0.06 μg/kg	
	Paprika			0.32 μg/kg	
	Coriander			0.31 μg/kg	
	Turmeric			1.9 μg/kg	
Malaysia	Dried chili, fennel, cumin, turmeric, black and white pepper, poppy seed, coriander, "garam masala," and mixed spices for fish, meat, and chicken curry	24	Total AFs/AFB1	Total AFs: 0.32-31.17 μg/kg AFB1: 0.32-28.43 μg/kg	[42]
Turkey	Red chili flake	24	Total AFs/AFB1/ AFB2	Total AF1: 3.09 μg/kg AFB1: 2.61 μg/kg AFB2: 0.24 μg/kg	[43]
	Red chili powder	22		Total AF1: 5.44 μg/kg AFB1: 5.10 μg/kg AFB2: 0.32 μg/kg	
	Black pepper powder	23		Total AF1: 0.24 μg/kg AFB1: 0.20 μg/kg AFB2: 0.05 μg/kg	
	Cumin	19		Total AF1: 0.62 μg/kg AFB1: 0.58 μg/kg AFB2: 0.08 μg/kg	

DOI: http://dx.doi.org/10.5772/intechopen.1009560

Country	Food product	Number of samples	Aflatoxin Types	Mean	References
Italy	Flour (all types)	90	AFB1	0.72 ± 1.00 μg/kg	[44]
	Wheat flour (conventional + organic)			—	
	Corn flour (conventional + organic)			0.72 ± 1.00 μg/kg	
	Conventional corn flour			0.85 ± 1.19 μg/kg	
	Organic corn flour			0.42 ± 0.43 μg/kg	
Turkey	Maize flour	24	AFB1	0.087-0.800 μg/kg	[45]
Iran	Wheat flour	200	Total AFs/AFB1/AFB2/AFG1/AFG2	Total AFs: 0.99 μg/kg AFB1: 0.53 μg/kg AFB2: 0.30 μg/kg AFG1: 0.55 μg/kg AFG2: 0.59 μg/kg	[46]

Table 2.
Global occurrence and levels of aflatoxins in various food products.

food safety concern. **Table 2** highlights significant variations in aflatoxin contamination levels across food products and countries across the world. For example, maize from the Democratic Republic of Congo showed some of the highest total aflatoxin levels, reaching up to 165.2 μg/kg, highlighting the risk of critical contamination in some regions for essential basic crops. Similarly, high levels of aflatoxin have been reported in peanuts from Pakistan (up to 7.30 μg/kg) and dried spices from Malaysia (up to 31.17 μg/kg), suggesting that post-harvest handling and storage conditions play a major role in contamination. In contrast, dairy products such as raw milk from Lebanon and Turkey showed relatively low levels of AFM1 (≤0.10437 μg/L).

4.2 Risk factors increasing aflatoxin contamination

As mentioned previously, aflatoxin contamination, mainly due to *A. flavus* and *A. parasiticus*, constitutes a major food safety concern due to its toxicity and carcinogenicity. There are different risk factors, including environmental, biological, and developmental influences that contribute to the prevalence and severity of aflatoxin contamination in agricultural crops and products.

4.2.1 Environmental factors

4.2.1.1 Temperature and water activity

The optimal temperature for aflatoxin production in *Aspergillus* species can differ slightly depending on the strain and substrate. However, in general, studies suggest that the optimum temperature range lies between 24 and 30°C [47]. Temperature effects can also depend on water activity, with some strains showing variation in optimal temperature based on the moisture content. It must be noted that high water activity (≥ 0.95) further enhances aflatoxin biosynthesis [19]. Therefore, the temperature range of 24-30°C is generally optimal, though it can vary slightly across different conditions [47]. Hence, environmental fluctuations outside of these parameters can often hinder toxin production but do not entirely prevent fungal growth [19].

4.2.1.2 Light exposure

Some studies reported the effect of light exposure on aflatoxin production. It was shown that darkness and low-light conditions can increase aflatoxin production, while light exposure can suppress its synthesis in some strains [47].

4.2.1.3 pH

pH is another important environmental factor that significantly impacts aflatoxin production. The transcription factor *pacC* plays a central role in the fungal response to pH changes [19, 47]. The *PacC* signaling pathway involves six additional proteins with Pal domains that sense and respond to pH shifts [19]. Studies show that the optimal pH range for aflatoxin production in *A. parasiticus* lies between 5 and 7 [47], suggesting that a slightly acidic to neutral environment is most favorable [24, 47].

4.2.2 Nutritional factors

4.2.2.1 Carbon sources

The type and availability of carbon sources play a critical role in aflatoxin production [19, 24, 47]. In *Aspergillus*, the sugar cluster near the aflatoxin (AF) gene cluster regulates carbon utilization. Carbon catabolic repression (CCR) allows *Aspergillus* to prioritize energy-efficient carbon sources through the transcription factor *CreA*, which influences genes associated with aflatoxin production. Although the genes in the aflatoxin pathway lack direct *CreA* binding sites and are not traditionally subject to carbon catabolite repression, *CreA* may still regulate *aflR* expression, indirectly affecting the levels of *AflR* protein. Additionally, *Rgt1*, a glucose-responsive regulator, might influence *aflJ*, which functions as a coactivator of *aflR* [19]. Certain sugars, such as sucrose, glucose, fructose, and sorbitol, are preferred for AFB1 production as they provide polyketide precursors like acetyl-CoA. However, some sugar derivatives, including D-glucal (which fungi cannot metabolize), and other sugars such as mannitol and galactose, inhibit AFB1 production [19, 47]. While glucose is the most efficient carbon source, aflatoxin synthesis can still occur using other carbon sources such as ribose, xylose, and glycerol. Several genes, including *creA, creB, alcR,* and *aldA,* are involved in carbon utilization in *Aspergillus* species [19].

4.2.2.2 Nitrogen sources

The variability among *Aspergillus* strains in response to nitrate, which can either inhibit or increase the aflatoxin biosynthetic pathway, has been linked to differences in the number of GATA sites near *aflJ*. This supports the role of these sites in environmental sensitivity [24]. Nitrate may influence aflatoxin gene expression by activating the *AreA* transcription factor; hence, it can regulate *aflR* and *aflJ*. However, the mechanism by which nitrate suppresses aflatoxin production remains unclear [24]. It is suggested that nitrate may suppress aflatoxin synthesis by increasing the NADPH/NADP ratio, which promotes fatty acid synthesis instead. The nitrogen source significantly impacts aflatoxin production in *Aspergillus* species [24]. Nitrogen sources such as casamino acids, asparagine, ammonium salts, glycine, and glutamate tend to enhance aflatoxin production. However, sodium nitrate, caffeine, and tryptophan do not have a similar effect [19, 47]. It must be noted that several genes, including *areA, nmrA, meaB,* and *niiA,* play important roles in nitrogen utilization in *Aspergillus* species [19].

4.2.2.3 Mineral availability

Micronutrients such as zinc play an essential role in enhancing aflatoxin synthesis. For example, in a synthetic media, the addition of 1-25 μg/mL zinc resulted in significantly increased toxin levels [47]. However, high levels of certain minerals, such as cadmium or mercury, can inhibit toxin production [47].

4.2.2.4 Lipid content in crops

The composition of crops, especially high lipid content, can also influence aflatoxin production. Lipids provide a rich energy source for fungal metabolism, therefore supporting aflatoxin biosynthesis. Crops rich in lipids, such as peanuts and other oilseeds, are particularly susceptible to contamination, as the availability of these substrates enhances fungal growth and toxin production [48].

4.2.3 Developmental and biological factors

The percentage of toxigenic isolates varies geographically and with the substrate [47]. Besides, aflatoxin production is influenced by factors like fungal species, plant stress from weeds, and insect damage [48]. In addition, sporulation is positively correlated with secondary metabolite production, including aflatoxins. Non-sporulating mutants exhibit reduced aflatoxin production. Additionally, the presence of smaller sclerotia ($\leq$400 μm) has been associated with higher aflatoxin levels, while larger sclerotia correlate with lower toxin levels [47].

4.3 Economic impact and regulatory standards for aflatoxins in food

Global agricultural trade suffers large financial losses due to aflatoxin contamination, especially affecting high-value commodities such as tree nuts, peanuts, and maize. From 2010 to 2019, aflatoxins above regulatory limits accounted for nearly 99% of U.S. mycotoxin warnings sent to the European Union's Rapid Alert System for Food and Feed (RASFF). The strict EU aflatoxin thresholds, which significantly impede U.S. exports, are reflected in these rejections, which mostly concern peanuts, pistachios, and almonds. The effects on the economy are considerably more noticeable for African countries. African exporters are estimated to lose $670 million in trade each year due to the EU's strict regulations, which are set at 2 μg/kg for AFB1 and 4 μg/kg for total aflatoxins. These limits mostly affect shipments of peanuts and maize [1, 49]. Besides, aflatoxin contamination causes major financial losses for the U.S. maize business as well. The costs are predicted to range from $52.1 million to $1.68 billion per year, depending on the extent of contamination and the climate. Reduced prices, returned shipments, and higher testing and compliance expenses are the causes of these losses. Additionally, the yearly costs of managing aflatoxin contamination in the U.S., including testing and mitigation techniques, range from $20 to $50 million. Farmers and grain handlers are further taxed by economic losses that can surpass $1 billion during years of increased contamination, such as drought years in the U.S. Corn Belt [49, 50].

Aflatoxin contamination has an impact on trade dynamics globally by requiring exporters to align with countries with comparable regulatory standards to prevent shipment rejections. Countries with strict limitations, such as the EU, impose significant financial penalties on exporters who do not comply, while countries with liberal or nonexistent aflatoxin rules frequently receive commodities with the greater levels of contamination [1, 49]. About 63% of the 4752 notifications of mycotoxin contamination in nuts and seeds that the EU received between 2011 and 2021 involved aflatoxins, highlighting the ongoing obstacles that such contamination poses to global trade [1, 49]. The economic tax on aflatoxins is worse with climatic fluctuation and regulatory obstacles. High temperatures and drought, like those that occurred in the Corn Belt in some years, raise the possibility of contamination and call for more regular testing. Due to varying contamination levels, these environmental conditions not only increase the risk of contamination but also increase economic losses, making it challenging for exporters to predict financial results [50]. Improved aflatoxin control measures, worldwide regulatory alignment, and cost-effective testing

Category	AFB1 (μg/kg)	Total AFs (AFB1 + AFB2 + AFG1 + AFG2) (μg/kg)
Groundnuts (direct consumption)	≤2	≤4
Groundnuts (before treatment)	≤8	≤15
Tree nuts (such as almonds and pistachios)	≤5-8	≤10
Cereals and derived products	≤2	≤4
Maize and rice (before treatment)	≤5	≤10
Dried fruits (direct consumption)	≤2	≤4
Dried figs	≤6	≤10
	AFM1 (μg/kg)	
Raw and heat-treated milk	≤0.05	

Table 3.
EU maximum limits for aflatoxins in food products [53].

technologies are urgently needed to decrease the financial taxes on global trade. This is highlighted by the combined effects of trade restrictions, management costs, and climatic variables.

Many countries have implemented regulations to protect consumers from the adverse effects of aflatoxins [51]. Various national and international organizations, such as the EU, the FDA, and the Food and Agriculture Organization (FAO), have tackled the aflatoxin issue by establishing a spectrum of standards, recommendations, and guidelines to regulate key aflatoxins in food products [1]. The FDA classifies human food with total aflatoxin levels above 20 ppb as unsafe and unsuitable for consumption [52]. By contrast, as shown in **Table 3,** the EU introduced a stricter and more detailed framework, with specific regulations set for aflatoxin B1 and total aflatoxins in various food categories, illustrating differences in food safety policies. For example, according to EU regulations, the maximum permitted level for AFB1 in peanuts intended for direct consumption is set at 2 μg/kg, and the total aflatoxin threshold must not exceed 4 μg/kg. In contrast, the FDA allows a significantly higher total aflatoxin threshold of 20 μg/kg for all food products, regardless of category. Similarly, while the EU limits the level of AFM1 in milk to 0.05 μg/kg, the FDA allows up to 0.5 μg/kg, a tenfold difference. This significant difference highlights different approaches to food safety. As the EU follows a precautionary approach, aiming to limit even minimal exposure to aflatoxins due to their carcinogenic risks, the FDA focuses on balancing safety with economic factors, possessing higher limits that may be more feasible for producers but could increase potential risks to consumers.

5. Health risks of AFB1 consumption in humans

Before discussing the adverse effects of AFB1 on human health, it is crucial to understand its absorption, metabolism, and excretion processes in the human body. AFB1 is primarily metabolized in the liver by cytochrome P450 (CYP450) enzymes, where the enzymes CYP1A2 and CYP3A4 are essential for its activation in the human liver [54, 55]. CYP1A2 converts AFM1 into AFM1 – 8, 9-epoxide, while CYP3A4 facilitates the conversion of AFB1 into AFB1-8,9 epoxide [55]. In addition, AFBO can undergo spontaneous hydrolysis to form AFB1 dihydrodiol, which may lead to tissue damage, inflammation, and excessive cell proliferation by binding to various proteins, ultimately contributing to carcinogenesis [55].

Moreover, AFB1 can produce various hydroxylated derivatives such as AFM1, AFQ1, AFP1, and AFL by its metabolism *via* P450 enzyme system. AFM1, a key metabolite, is excreted in milk and urine, and its levels correlate with AFB1 exposure. Unlike AFB1, AFM1 demonstrates direct cytotoxicity without requiring metabolic activation in the liver, as seen in human intestinal cells (Caco-2) and other cell lines. This cytotoxicity involves reactive oxygen species (ROS) production [6].

5.1 Carcinogenic mechanisms of AFB1

5.1.1 Activation of AhR pathway

The activation of this pathway starts when the *AhR* receptor detects toxic compounds like aflatoxins and helps to detoxify them. The first step includes the binding of harmful chemicals called ligands like aflatoxins to AhR receptors, present in the cytoplasm [56]. This binding causes a change in the confirmation of the PAS A domain present in the AhR receptor. AhR receptor dissociates then from Hsp90 proteins and moves into the nucleus by a process mediated by importins. Inside the nucleus, *AhR* pairs with another protein called Arnt, and they form together a functional complex [56]. The *AhR-Arnt* complex binds to specific DNA sequences in the promoter target genes called AhR Response Elements (ARES) [57]. The target genes include CYP1A1, CYP1A2, and CYP1B1, which produce enzymes crucial for the metabolic activation of AFB1 into more reactive forms that can cause DNA damage [57]. *AhR* causes an up-regulation of these cytochrome P450 Phase 1 hydroxylases (CYP1A1, CYP1A2, CYP1B1) and the conversion of the parent pro-carcinogen into mutagenic epoxide intermediates through biotransformation [58]. However, mice deficient in these hydroxylases were found to have a reduced incidence of malignant lymphomas and other tumors, such as those induced by PAHs [58].

The *AhR*, which is inactive in its resting state, can be activated by environmental chemicals (ligands) to trigger the production of Phase 1 P450 hydroxylases. These enzymes create harmful intermediates from pro-carcinogen compounds or certain natural substances (like estradiol or polyunsaturated fats), which can mutate DNA and lead to cancer [58]. In addition to its overexpression, the *AhR* seems to be constantly active in various types of human cancers, including glioblastomas, adult T cell leukemias, as well as breast, oral, lung, liver, and prostate adenocarcinomas [59]. An elevated *AhR* expression and activity was typically associated with increased levels of *AhR* target genes such as CYP1A1 and CYP1B1 in cancers of the gastrointestinal tract, bladder, head and neck, and breast [58].

Due to its planar structure of AFB1 similar to that of the known ligands, it can act as an activator of the *AhR*. Thus, it binds to the *AhR* receptor and triggers its translocation to the nucleus. Its ability to activate transcriptional expression of CYP1A1 in H4IIE hepatoma cells suggests it may act as an agonist for the *AhR*, although direct evidence is still lacking [4]. This suggests that activation of the *AhR* pathway may be a mechanism underlying AFB1 toxicity [4]. The activation of *AhR* by AFB1 leads to the induction of free radicals and reactive oxygen species (ROS), which are thought to play a key role in carcinogenesis and the progression of carcinomas [4]. This process can reduce immune surveillance of carcinogenesis by affecting the regulatory function of T CD4+ lymphocytes [60]. AFB1 binding to *AhR* triggers a rapid response involving the activation of tyrosine kinases, as well as the ERK and PKC1 signaling pathways that can contribute to

DOI: http://dx.doi.org/10.5772/intechopen.1009560

cancer development. In human hepatocyte cultures, AFB1 also increases the transcriptional expression of RXR and enhances the expression of CYP2B6 and CYP3A5 cytochrome genes, which are regulated by this receptor [57].

5.1.2 Alteration of non-coding RNAs (miRNA) expression

MicroRNAs (miRNAs) are small non-coding RNA molecules regulating gene expression by binding to complementary sequences within target mRNAs. They play critical roles in regulating the toxic and carcinogenic effects of AFB1, particularly in liver cancer [3]. Many analyses showed that AFs-regulated miRNAs impact pathways such as *p53* signaling, cell cycle, Wnt signaling, and JAK/STAT signaling [3]. For instance, elevated levels of miR-33a and miR-34a suppressed the Wnt/β-catenin signaling pathway in HCC cells exposed to AFB1 [55]. Aflatoxins have been shown to influence miRNA expression, upregulating molecules such as miR-34a-5p, miR-33a-5p, and miR-122-5p in various models [3, 55]. Studies on F344 rats exposed to AFB1 for 4 weeks showed significant upregulation of miR-122-5p, miR-34a-5p, and miR-181c-3p in liver tissue and blood during the early stages of carcinogenesis, highlighting AFB1-induced epigenetic changes [6]. In addition, key microRNAs such as miR-429 and miR-24 are upregulated in AFB1-exposed liver cancer tissues, increasing the formation of AFB1-DNA adduct, and inhibiting apoptosis, which makes them considered reliable biomarkers for AFB1-induced liver cancer [55]. These findings suggest AFs significantly alter miRNA expression and related biological processes, contributing to their cytotoxic and carcinogenic effects.

5.1.3 DNA damage

Several steps of AFB1 oxidation result in two isomers: AFB1-endo-8,9 epoxide and AFB1-exo-8,9-epoxide (AFBO). Compared to the endo-isomer, AFBO is the most reactive, unstable, and toxic of the two isomers, with the endo-isomer considered less reactive and less toxic by comparison [61]. Once exo-AFBO is formed, it binds to the N^7 atom of guanine residues and forms AFB1-N^7-guanine adducts, causing mutations that can lead to carcinogenesis [54, 55, 61]. The resulting AFB1-N^7-guanine adduct can follow two pathways:

- Under alkaline conditions, AFB1-N^7-guanine dissociates from the DNA forming an open ring, which leads to the formation of cis- and trans-AFB1 formamidopyrimidine adducts, known as minor and major AFB1-FAPy adducts [54, 55, 61]. The higher mutagenicity of AFB1-FAPy lesions is complex and cannot be solely attributed to their resistance to repair by the Nucleotide Excision Repair (NER) system [61].

- Compared to the AFB1-N^7-guanine adduct, AFB1-FAPy adducts exhibit a shorter elimination half-life [6]. They can undergo spontaneous depurination, leaving an abasic (AP) site in the DNA backbone. These AP sites, which are endogenous, can be quickly repaired while releasing free AFB1-N^7-guanine. AP sites caused by depurination are common mutation-promoting lesions, with an estimated 30,000 AP sites per cell being continuously present [6].

Both AP sites and AFB1-FAPy lesions act as precursors to gene mutations, with the specific location of these mutations influencing whether cancer development is initiated [6]. The AFB1-N^7-guanine adduct exhibited a mutagenic efficiency of 45% in COS-7 cells (kidney cell line) [62]. This indicated that 45% of these adducts induced measurable mutations in the transfected plasmid. The primary mutation observed was a G:C to T:A base pair substitution. In comparison, the AFB1-FAPy adducts demonstrated a significantly higher mutagenic efficiency of 97% in the same *in vitro* system highlighting its strong mutagenic potential [62].

5.1.4 p53 gene mutation

One of the major mutations caused by AFBO following exposure to AFB1 is a transversion mutation that occurs in the *p53* gene. This mutation replaces guanine (G) with thymine (T) at codon 249 of the *p53* gene, resulting in the substitution of ^{249} Arg protein with ^{249} Ser protein [6]. Codon 249, particularly guanine nucleotide, is considered a mutation hotspot frequently detected in liver cancer patients from regions with high AFB1 exposure [6]. These mutations in the *p53* gene result in its loss of function, leading to dysregulation of critical cellular processes such as cell cycle control, DNA repair, and apoptosis.

The loss of *p53* function results in the absence of *p21*, a protein regulated by *p53*, leading to uncontrolled CDK activity and preventing the formation of the DREAM complex. The DREAM complex, composed of DP, RB-like, E2F, and MuvB, is essential for the regulation of the cell cycle by repressing the transcription of genes essential for its progression [61, 63]. Without the formation of DREAM complex, transcriptional activators bind to E2F and CHR promoters, driving the expression of genes such as PLK1, cyclins, and CDC proteins that promote cell cycle progression. Consequently, this prevents the cell cycle arrest at critical checkpoints [61, 63]. Under normal conditions, *p21* interacts with proliferating cell nuclear antigen (PCNA) to prevent its association with DNA polymerase which inhibits DNA replication and repair. Loss of *p21* function disrupts this regulatory mechanism, leading to impaired DNA replication and repair [61].

In addition, the cytoplasmic localization of *p21* inhibits apoptotic enzymes such as ASK1, SAPK, and caspases, as well as transcription factors such as E2F1 and STAT3, thereby preventing the activation of pro-apoptotic genes [61]. This inhibition complements the loss of p53 function, as both mechanisms contribute to the suppression of apoptosis. *p53* typically upregulates *PUMA*, a pro-apoptotic protein that blocks pro-survival *Bcl-2* family proteins (e.g., *Bcl-2, Bcl-XL*). Without *p53* activity, *PUMA* expression is reduced, leaving these proteins active and inhibiting apoptosis by preventing mitochondrial damage and cytochrome C release [61].

5.1.5 Hepatocellular carcinoma (HCC)

Many studies have shown a strong link between AFB1 exposure and an increased risk of liver cancer. Furthermore, co-infection with HBV significantly amplifies this risk, increasing the likelihood of HCC by 30-fold in individuals exposed to AFB1 [61]. The *p53* tumor suppressor protein is frequently mutated in HCC. In regions with high AFB1 exposure, mutations in the *p53* gene at codon 249 are detected in 40% of patients with AFB1-associated hepatocarcinoma. In contrast, this mutation is rarely found in patients from areas with lower AFB1 exposure [64]. This ^{249}Ser mutation in the *p53* gene inhibits wild-type *p53* activity, promoting cell growth and survival. Additionally, AFB1-induced mutations in the *ras* oncogene and overexpression of the *c-fos* oncogene further contribute to liver cancer initiation [61]. In addition, AFB1 exposure alters methylation patterns of critical genes, including *RUNX3*, *LINE-1*, *CXCR4*, and *INTS1*, resulting in increased DNA damage and impaired cellular regulation. The dysregulated expression of genes such as *CCNK*, *PCNA*, and *TXNRD1* has been identified as potential early markers of AFB1-related HCC [61]. These molecular alterations underscore the significant role of AFB1 in initiating and promoting hepatocarcinogenesis through both genetic and epigenetic mechanisms.

On the other hand, the co-infection with HBV or HCV and exposure to aflatoxins can significantly amplify the risk of HCC by combining their individual carcinogenic effects [65]. The presence of HBV surface antigen (HBsAg) and AFs raises the risk of HCC by up to 60-fold. HBV and AFs enhance HCC development through various mechanisms: HBV prolongs the persistence of aflatoxin-DNA adducts, impairs hepatocyte metabolism of AFs, and increases oxidative stress, while AFs suppress cell-mediated immunity, facilitating HBV persistence and tumorigenesis [65]. The HBV-encoded HBx protein, or hepatitis B virus X protein, is a multifunctional regulatory protein encoded by the *HBx* gene of the HBV. It facilitates cell cycle progression, enhances telomerase reverse transcriptase expression, suppresses negative growth regulators, and interferes with the activity of tumor suppressor genes like *p53*, along with senescence-related factors, to inhibit apoptosis [65]. This synergistic interaction is more prevalent in resource-limited regions like sub-Saharan Africa and Asia, where exposure to AF-contaminated food and chronic HBV infection are common [65]. Epidemiological studies show that HBV amplifies the carcinogenic effects of AFs by promoting necro-inflammatory liver damage, increasing hepatocyte proliferation, and facilitating mutations like ^{249}Ser [66].

The synergistic effect of chronic HCV infection and aflatoxin exposure significantly enhances the risk of HCC due to their combined impact on liver damage and tumorigenesis. The viral core proteins, particularly NS3 and NS5A, which are non-structural proteins primarily associated with HCV, induce oxidative stress and activate pro-inflammatory and proliferative signaling pathways, contributing to DNA damage, cell death, and chronic liver injury [65]. HCV infection further amplifies the carcinogenic effects of aflatoxins by increasing oxidative stress and inflammation, thereby facilitating the formation of AFB1-DNA adducts and their persistence in hepatocytes [65]. In regions with high aflatoxin exposure and HCV prevalence, such as sub-Saharan Africa and parts of Asia, this synergism poses a significant public health threat. Epidemiological evidence highlights that individuals with chronic HCV infection who are exposed to aflatoxins have a markedly higher risk of developing HCC than those exposed to either factor alone [65].

5.2 Toxicity of AFB1

5.2.1 Hepatotoxicity

Caveolin-1 (*CAV1*) plays a central role in AFB1-induced hepatotoxicity by mediating key cellular processes such as oxidative stress and autophagy. In the human hepatocyte L02 cell line, AFB1 exposure leads to a significant increase in *CAV1* expression [55]. *CAV1* promotes oxidative stress through its interaction with *Nrf2*, which in turn reduces cellular antioxidant enzyme levels and activates apoptotic pathways in hepatocytes [55].

Aflatoxins disrupt mitochondrial function, triggering multiple cellular injury pathways. This disruption begins with mitochondrial damage and impairment. Under normal conditions, the mitochondria in hepatocytes are responsible for consuming about 90% of oxygen and performing oxidative phosphorylation (OXPHOS). In addition, *Bcl-2* prevents mitochondrial outer membrane permeabilization (MOMP) by its binding to activated *Bax* [61]. Exposure to aflatoxins and their metabolites leads to an impairment of mitochondrial respiratory chain complexes I-IV, which are crucial for electron transfer and ATP production. Aflatoxins also inhibit enzymes such as succinate dehydrogenase (SDH) and ATPase, resulting in a decrease in ATP synthesis and the mitochondrial respiratory control ratio (RCR) [61]. On the other hand, aflatoxins cause a reduction in *Bcl-2* levels, which leads to *Bax* activation, mitochondrial membrane disruption, and cytochrome c release. The increase of *Bax* expression is associated with a decrease in *Bcl-2/Bax* ratio, indicating apoptosis in hepatocytes [61, 67]. Furthermore, aflatoxins induce the opening of mitochondrial permeability transition pore (mPTP), leading to mitochondrial membrane damage and the release of enzymes such as ALT and AST into the serum [61]. AFB1 specifically induces *COX2* expression, promotes mitochondrial autophagy, and impairs mitochondrial lipid metabolism in hepatocytes [55].

The second disruption in hepatocyte mitochondria caused by aflatoxins is the excessive generation of reactive oxygen species (ROS), further amplifying oxidative stress and cellular damage. AFB1-induced ROS production activates the Keap1/Nrf2/ARE pathway, which modulates the expression of antioxidant genes like GPx4 to mitigate lipid peroxidation. However, lipid peroxides, including 4-hydroxylnonenal, disrupt membrane integrity and induce cytotoxicity, genotoxicity, and COX-2 expression, contributing to further cellular injury. This cascade highlights the multifaceted role of oxidative stress in AFs-induced hepatotoxicity [3].

When the mitochondrial damage caused by aflatoxins and the structural integrity of hepatocytes exceed the cell's repair mechanisms, hepatocytes trigger apoptosis to preserve normal liver function. However, this also results in hepatotoxicity [3]. Both the intrinsic and extrinsic apoptosis pathways contribute to hepatotoxicity by activating caspases, which cleave various intracellular substrates [3]. *In vitro* studies demonstrate that AFB1 induces hepatocyte apoptosis through both the mitochondrial and death receptor pathways [68].

Aflatoxins activate the intrinsic apoptosis pathway primarily through the opening of the mPTP. This process leads to swollen mitochondria and the collapse of the mitochondrial membrane potential (MMP), which releases electrons, cyt c, and other small molecules into the cytosol. The leakage of cyt c activates the formation of the apoptosome complex, which includes apoptotic protease-activating factor-1 (*Apaf-1*), cyt c, and *caspase-9*. This cascade leads to the activation and upregulation of caspase [3, 55].

The extrinsic cell death pathway is primarily initiated by the interaction between death receptors and their ligands, which play a crucial role in triggering apoptosis [3, 68]. In the liver, death receptors such as *Fas*, tumor necrosis factor receptor 1 (TNFR1*)*, and tumor necrosis factor-related apoptosis-inducing ligand receptors 1 and 2 (TRAIL-R1 and TRAIL-R2*)* recognize specific cytokines. TNFR1 interacts with death domain-associated proteins, including TNFR-associated protein with death *domain (TRADD),* TNF-associated factor-2 (TRAF2), and receptor-interacting protein (RIP) [3]. Aflatoxins lead to the upregulation of receptors such as *TNFR1* and *Fas,* which subsequently trigger apoptosis in hepatocytes through the death receptor pathway. AFs also increase the expression of TRADD and TRAF2 [3]. Upon receptor activation and oligomerization, caspase-8 and/or caspase-10 are cleaved, activating downstream caspases, such as caspase-3, caspase-6, and caspase-7, which are crucial for apoptosis. The expression of caspase-8 and caspase-10 increases also. Activated caspase-8 then initiates apoptosis through two pathways: by directly cleaving caspase-3 and by activating the pro-apoptotic *Bcl-2* family protein Bid. Bid triggers the release of cytochrome c from mitochondria, which activates *caspase-9*, further amplifying the apoptotic signal [3, 68].

Both the intrinsic and extrinsic pathways culminate in the activation of intracellular proteases and endonucleases that degrade cellular components. In conclusion, AFs impair hepatocyte function and structure by activating various cell death pathways, while inhibiting protective mechanisms, thereby exacerbating hepatotoxicity.

5.2.2 Immunotoxicity

AFB1 consumption significantly influences human immune function, affecting both the innate and adaptive immune systems [69]. This immunotoxic effect is mainly due to the reactive metabolite AFB1-exo-8,9-epoxide (AFBO), which interacts with immune cells, inhibiting their ability to proliferate and produce crucial immune responses [69]. Therefore, individuals exposed to AFB1 have increased susceptibility to infectious diseases, delayed recovery, and reduced vaccine efficacy [61]. In addition to these broader immune system disruptions, AFB1 also alters cytokine production, reducing interleukin-4 (IL-4) levels while enhancing the expression of pro-inflammatory cytokines such as interferon-γ (INFγ) and tumor necrosis factor-alpha (TNFα), further provoking immune system imbalances. In addition, exposure to AFB1 results in decreased levels of activated lymphocytes, impairing lymphoblastogenesis and the body's ability to induce delayed hypersensitivity responses, both crucial for defense against infections. Besides, it reduces levels of immunoglobulins (IgM, IgA, and IgG), thereby increasing the risk of infections [69] . *In vitro* studies have shown that AFB1 inhibits the multiplication of human lymphocytes with high concentrations leading to a significant increase in both apoptotic and necrotic lymphocytes, further impairing immune functions [61]. Cellular immunity is particularly sensitive to the effects of AFB1, being more severely affected compared to humoral immunity, indicating that the body's ability to fight infections is significantly reduced [61, 69].

5.2.3 Other types of toxicity

AFB1 also exhibits a range of other toxic effects. These effects affect different organ systems, leading to major health complications through distinct mechanisms. **Table 4** discusses these less-discussed toxicities, focusing on enterotoxicity, nephrotoxicity, neurotoxicity, and reproductive toxicity. Each category highlights key mechanisms, effects, and conclusions to provide a comprehensive understanding of the broader toxicological impact of AFB1 (**Table 4**) [55].

5.3 Oxidative stress

Aflatoxins cause oxidative stress by targeting mitochondria, which are the primary site of cellular energy production and ROS generation. These toxins affect mitochondrial respiratory chain complexes (I-IV), leading to disruption of electron transport and decreased ATP synthesis, which includes cellular energy metabolism. Simultaneously, electron leakage from damaged complexes intensifies the production of ROS, including superoxide radicals, thereby provoking oxidative stress [3]. The imbalance is further intensified as FAs decrease key antioxidant defenses, including manganese superoxide dismutase (Mn-SOD), glutathione peroxidase (GPx), and catalase (CAT), while depleting

Type of toxicity	Mechanism	Effect	Key findings
Enterotoxicity	Disruption of intestinal barrier function, damage to epithelial cells, and alteration of gut microbiota	Chronic intestinal diseases, reduced nutrient absorption, metabolic dysfunction	Damage of intestinal villi, reduction of height and density, alteration of gut microbiota similar to inflammatory bowel disease (IBD) patients.
Nephrotoxicity	AFB1 accumulation in renal tissue, oxidative stress, upregulation of *p21*, and mitochondrial dysfunction	Apoptosis, renal tissue damage, synergistic effects with other toxins	Promotes oxidative stress, S-phase arrest, and DNA fragmentation in renal cells, exacerbating renal dysfunction under low-protein diets
Neurotoxicity	Penetration of blood-brain barrier, neuroinflammation, mitochondrial dysfunction, and induction of neuronal apoptosis	Impaired brain function, chronic neurodegenerative conditions (such as Alzheimer's symptoms)	Observed pathological changes in cerebral cortex and hippocampus, increased susceptibility to neurodegenerative diseases
Reproductive toxicity	Oxidative stress and DNA damage disrupting gametogenesis, spermatogenesis, and embryonic development	Reduced gamete quality, impaired spermatogenesis, oocyte damage, testicular dysfunction, and fetal health issues	Crosses placental barrier and affects embryo development and sperm DNA integrity

Table 4.
Overview of other types of toxic effects of AFB1 on human health [55].

glutathione (GSH), a crucial coenzyme for neutralizing ROS. Also, high levels of ROS trigger lipid peroxidation, leading to membrane damage, altered fluidity, and increased permeability [3]. Additionally, hydrogen peroxide generated during oxidative processes intervenes in the Fenton reaction, creating hydroxyl radicals that further make the cellular damage worse. Together, these processes generate a feedback cycle of mitochondrial dysfunction and ROS production, intensifying oxidative stress and its detrimental consequences on cellular integrity [3].

Activation of the oxidative stress signaling pathways, particularly the *Nrf2* pathway, is a crucial mechanism in AFB1-induced hepatotoxicity. Under normal physiological conditions, *Nrf2* is retained in the cytoplasm by its inhibitor Keap1 (Kelch-like ECH—ECH-associated protein) and undergoes degradation [67, 68]. However, in response to the oxidative stress, *Nrf2* dissociates from *Keap1*. It translocates to the nucleus, where it binds to antioxidant response elements (AREs) in DNA, thereby activating the expression of detoxifying and antioxidant genes [67, 68]. These genes encode enzymes such as heme oxygenase-1 (HO-1), glutathione S-transferase, and NAD (P)H quinone oxidoreductase, which together contribute to reducing the oxidative damage [55, 67, 68]. It must be noted that AFB1 significantly disrupts this pathway by inhibiting *Nrf2* expression and decreasing HO-1 levels. This elimination provokes oxidative stress, contributing to lipid peroxidation and DNA damage. Moreover, the interaction of AFB1 with the *Nrf2* pathway is linked to other signaling cascades, such as NF-KB, which is linked to inflammation, and mTOR, which controls autophagy, thereby enhancing liver toxicity [55, 68]. In general, some phytochemicals show the protective effects by stimulating *Nrf2* activation. However, the persistent inhibition of the pathway by AFB1 underlines its complex role in the regulation of oxidative stress and liver damage [67, 68].

5.4 Inflammation

Aflatoxins activate the NF-κB pathway, leading to the overexpression of pro-inflammatory cytokines such as TNF-α, IL-1β, IL-6, and IL-8, which contribute to systemic inflammation [70]. In addition, aflatoxins trigger the upregulation of the *NLRP3* inflammasome pathway, further increasing the release of these pro-inflammatory cytokines [71]. When food-borne aflatoxins enter the body, they cause inflammation in the cells, and the liver is equally affected [72]. Nuclear factor NF-kappa B (NF-KB) has been extensively researched because it is a major inflammatory factor in the majority of inflammatory reactions. Aflatoxins-induced liver inflammation is closely linked to NF-KB activation, according to recent research [67]. HepG2 cells, piglets, and OTA were used to create liver injury models using AFB1, OTA, DON, and ZEN, respectively. This suggests that these four food-borne mycotoxins including AFB1 can cause severe liver inflammation by activating the classical inflammatory pathway NF-KB and up-regulating inflammatory cytokines such as Interleukin1b (IL-1b), Interleukin-8 (IL-8), TNF-α, and COX-2 [73, 74]. Numerous studies have shown that AFB1 increases the level of inflammatory cytokines in mouse livers; however, it is still unknown whether the NF-KB pathway is activated in AFB1-induced liver inflammation. The primary mechanism of hepatotoxicity caused by AFB1 is that it inhibits the liver's production of ceramide synthase, activates sphingolipid metabolism, causes sphingosine accumulation, and triggers a strong inflammatory reaction [75, 76].

As a molecular platform, the *NLRP3* assembly creates the *NLRP3* inflammasome, a large cytosolic protein complex that triggers the self-cleavage and activation of the cysteine protease caspase-1, transforming pro-IL-1β and pro-IL-18 into their mature forms. Initiation and activation are the two sequential steps needed to activate the *NLRP3* inflammasome [77]. The first step involves TLR recognizing DAMPs, which causes NF-κB to become activated, pro-IL-1β to be inducted, and NLRP3 synthesis to increase. Different extracellular stimuli cause the inflammasome complex to assemble and ultimately become activated during the activation step [3]. NOD-, LRR-, and pyrin domain-containing protein 3 (*NLRP3*) is a sensor of intracellular inflammation. The *NLRP3* inflammasome is a cytosolic multiprotein complex generated of a sensor (*NLRP3*), an adaptor (ASC), and an effector (caspase 1) [78]. The formation of the *NLRP3* inflammasome may cause the pro-inflammatory cytokines IL-1β and IL-18 to be released caspase 1-dependently, as well as encourage gasdermin D-mediated pyroptotic cell death. During cell pyroptosis, Gasdermin D (GSDMD) is typically cleaved by caspase-11 or caspase-1 to produce a 31 kDa N-terminal fragment (e.g., GSDMD-N) [79]. In primary mouse microglia, exposure to AFB1 and AFM1 markedly enhanced the expression of *NLRP3*, caspase-1 and GSDMD-N, and ASC proteins [78]. Dimethyl fumarate's inhibition of GSDMD significantly decreased the inflammatory response and cell pyroptosis in microglial cells produced by AFB1 and AFM1. These investigations demonstrate that AFB1-induced neurotoxicity is facilitated by cell pyroptosis and the NLRP3 inflammasome-mediated response [80].

6. Conclusion

Aflatoxins, particularly AFB1, pose a major global health hazard due to their widespread presence in food and feed and their potent toxic and carcinogenic effects. Understanding the production and potential contamination of crops by these toxins requires the study of their biochemistry and biosynthesis, which are influenced by both genetic factors and environmental conditions. The economic impact of aflatoxin contamination, particularly in crops such as maize and peanuts, highlights the need for effective preventive strategies. The health hazards associated with aflatoxins, such as hepatotoxicity, carcinogenicity, oxidative stress, and apoptosis, emphasize the critical importance of treating exposure to these toxins. Advances in genetic engineering, the use of natural inhibitors, and antifungal agents present potential options to decrease aflatoxin production, but challenges persist in effectively implementing these solutions. Regulatory limits set by agencies such as the EU and FDA are crucial to managing exposure, but continued research into the molecular mechanisms of aflatoxin toxicity and prevention is essential. Eventually, solving the global aflatoxin problem requires a comprehensive approach that includes improved detection methods, better agricultural practices, and continued innovation in biotechnology, coupled with the strict regulatory measures to protect public health.

Nomenclature

AF	Aflatoxin
EU	European Union
U.S.	United States
FDA	Food and Drug Administration
SSA	Sub-Saharan Africa
HCC	Hepatocellular carcinoma
DNA	Deoxyribonucleic acid
HIV	Human immunodeficiency virus
kb	Kilobases
A. flavus	*Aspergillus flavus*
A. parasiticus	*Aspergillus parasiticus*
NOR	Norsoloric acid
NAA	Norsolorinic acid anthrone
VAA	Versicolorin
AVN	Averantin
HAVN	Hydroxyaverantin
OAVN	Oxoaverantin
AVF	Averufin
DMST	Demethylsterigmatocystin
ST	Sterigmatocystin
OMST	O-methylsterigmatocystin
NADP	Nicotinamide adenine dinucleotide phosphate
AMP	Adenosine monophosphate
CCR	Carbon catabolic repression
RASFF	Rapid Alert System for Food and Feed
CYP450	Cytochrome P450
ROS	Reactive oxygen species
ARES	AhR response elements
PAHs	Polycyclic aromatic hydrocarbons
H4IIE	Rat hepatoma cell line
AFBO	AFB1-endo-8,9 epoxide/AFB1-exo-8,9 epoxide
NER	Nucleotide Excision Repair
AP	Abasic

COS-7 cells	Kidney cell line
Arg protein	Arginine protein
Ser protein	Serine protein
CDK	Cyclin-dependent kinase
DREAM	DP, RB-like, E2F, and MuvB complex
CDC	Cell division cycle
HBV	Hepatitis B virus
HCV	Hepatitis C virus
HBsAg	HBV surface antigen
CAV1	Caveolin-1
OXPHOS	Oxidative phosphorylation
MOMP	Mitochondrial outer membrane permeability
ATP	Adenosine triphosphate
SDH	Succinate dehydrogenase
RCR	Respiratory control ratio
MMP	Mitochondrial membrane potential
Apaf-1	Apoptotic protease-activating factor-1
TNFR1	Tumor necrosis factor receptor 1
TRAIL-R1 and TRAIL-R2	Tumor necrosis factor-related apoptosis-including ligand receptors 1 and 2
TRADD	TNFR-associated protein with death domain
RIP	Receptor-interacting protein
IL	Interleukin
INFγ	Interferon-γ
TNFα	Tumor necrosis factor-α
Ig	Immunoglobulin
IBD	Inflammatory bowel disease
Mn-SOD	Manganese-superoxide dismutase
GSH	Glutathione
GPx	Glutathione peroxidase
CAT	Catalase
Keapl	Kelch-like ECH-ECH-associated protein
HO-1	Heme oxygenase-1
HepG2	Human hepatocellular carcinoma cell line
OTA	Ochratoxin A
DON	Deoxynivalenol
ZEN	Zearalenone
NF-KB	Nuclear factor NF-kappa B
COX-2	Cyclooxygenase-2
NLRP3	NOD-, LRR-, and pyrin domain-containing protein 3
GSDMD	Gasdermin D

Author details

Heba Hellany[1†], Rayan Kashmar[2,3†], Ghosoon Albahri[3] and Jean-Claude Assaf[4*]

1 Department of Biology, American University of Beirut, Beirut, Lebanon

2 IMT Atlantique, Energy Systems and Environment Department, GEPEA, Rue Alfred Kastler, France

3 Doctoral School of Science and Technology, Research and Analysis Platform in Environmental Sciences (EDST-PRASE), Beirut, Lebanon

4 Microbial Engineering Laboratory, Department of Chemical Engineering, Faculty of Engineering, University of Balamand, Tripoli, Lebanon

*Address all correspondence to: jeanclaude.assaf@balamand.edu.lb

† These authors contributed equally.

References

[1] Hellany H, Assaf JC, El-Badan D, Khalil M. Quantification, prevalence, and Pretreatment methods of mycotoxins in groundnuts and tree nuts: An update. Processes. 2023;**11**(12):3428

[2] Ferreira RG, Cardoso MV, De Souza Furtado KM, Espíndola KMM, Amorim RP, Monteiro MC. Epigenetic alterations caused by aflatoxin B1: A public health risk in the induction of hepatocellular carcinoma. Translational Research. 2019;**204**:51-71

[3] Hua Z, Liu R, Chen Y, Liu G, Li C, Song Y, et al. Contamination of aflatoxins induces severe hepatotoxicity through multiple mechanisms. Frontiers in Pharmacology. 2021;**11**:605823

[4] Mary VS, Valdehita A, Navas JM, Rubinstein HR, Fernández-Cruz ML. Effects of aflatoxin B1, fumonisin B1 and their mixture on the aryl hydrocarbon receptor and cytochrome P450 1A induction. Food and Chemical Toxicology. 2015;**75**:104-111

[5] Amare MG, Keller NP. Molecular mechanisms of aspergillus flavus secondary metabolism and development. Fungal Genetics and Biology. 2014;**66**:11-18

[6] Cao W, Yu P, Yang K, Cao D. Aflatoxin B1: Metabolism, toxicology, and its involvement in oxidative stress and cancer development. Toxicology Mechanisms and Methods. 2022;**32**(6):395-419. DOI: 10.1080/15376516.2021.2021339

[7] Benkerroum N. Aflatoxins: Producing-molds, structure, health issues and incidence in Southeast Asian and Sub-Saharan African countries. International Journal of Environmental Research and Public Health [Internet]. 2020;**17**(4):1215. Available from: https://www.mdpi.com/1660-4601/17/4/1215

[8] Liu Yan W, Felicia. Global burden of aflatoxin-induced hepatocellular carcinoma: A risk assessment. Environmental Health Perspectives [Internet]. 2010;**118**(6):818-824. DOI: 10.1289/ehp.0901388

[9] Benkerroum N. Mycotoxins in dairy products: A review. International Dairy Journal [Internet]. 2016;**62**:63-75 Available from: https://linkinghub.elsevier.com/retrieve/pii/S095869461630214X

[10] Wogan GN. Chemical nature and biological effects of the aflatoxins. Bacteriological Reviews [Internet]. 1966;**30**(2):460-470. DOI: 10.1128/br.30.2.460-470.1966

[11] Cole RJ, Kirksey JW. Aflatoxin G1 metabolism by Rhizopus species. Journal of Agricultural and Food Chemistry [Internet]. 1971;**19**(2):222-223. DOI: 10.1021/jf60174a044

[12] Abrehame S, Manoj VR, Hailu M, Chen YY, Lin YC, Chen YP. Aflatoxins: Source, detection, clinical features and prevention. Processes [Internet]. 2023;**11**(1):204. Available from: https://www.mdpi.com/2227-9717/11/1/204

[13] Dilkin P, Zorzete P, Mallmann CA, Gomes JDF, Utiyama CE, Oetting LL, et al. Toxicological effects of chronic low doses of aflatoxin B1 and fumonisin B1-containing Fusarium moniliforme culture material in weaned piglets. Food and Chemical Toxicology [Internet]. 2003;**41**(10):1345-1353. Available from: https://linkinghub.elsevier.com/retrieve/pii/S0278691503001376

[14] World Health Organization, Food and Agriculture Organization of the United Nations, Joint FAO/WHO Expert Committee on Food Additives. Meeting (72nd): 2010 : Rome I. Evaluation of Certain Contaminants in Food: Seventy-Second [72nd] Report of the Joint FAO/WHO Expert Committee on Food Additives. WHO; 2011. p. 105. Available from: https://iris.who.int/handle/10665/44514

[15] Wong JJ, Hsieh DP. Mutagenicity of aflatoxins related to their metabolism and carcinogenic potential. Proceedings of the National Academy of Sciences of the United States of America. [Internet]. 1976;**73**(7):2241-2244. DOI: 10.1073/pnas.73.7.2241

[16] Hellany H, Assaf JC, Matta J, Khalil MI. Fungal isolation, detection, and quantification of aflatoxins in nuts sold in the Lebanese market. Processes. 2024;**12**(5):1018

[17] Williams JH, Phillips TD, Jolly PE, Stiles JK, Jolly CM, Aggarwal D. Human aflatoxicosis in developing countries: A review of toxicology, exposure, potential health consequences, and interventions. The American Journal of Clinical Nutrition. 2004;**80**(5):1106-1122. Available from: https://linkinghub.elsevier.com/retrieve/pii/S000291652203667X

[18] Horn BW. Ecology and population biology of Aflatoxigenic fungi in soil. Journal of Toxicology: Toxin Reviews. 2003;**22**(2-3):351-379

[19] Caceres I, Al Khoury A, El Khoury R, Lorber S, Oswald PI, El Khoury A, et al. Aflatoxin biosynthesis and genetic regulation: A review. Toxins. 2020;**12**(3):150

[20] Khan R, Ghazali FM, Mahyudin NA, Samsudin NIP. Updates on the functions and molecular mechanisms of the genes involved in aspergillus flavus development and biosynthesis of aflatoxins. Journal of Fungi. 2021;7(8):606

[21] Khan R, Ghazali FM, Mahyudin NA, Samsudin NIP. Aflatoxin biosynthesis, genetic regulation, toxicity, and control strategies: A review. Journal of Fungi. 2021;7(8):606

[22] Mejia-Teniente L, Maria A, Alejandro M, Torres-Pacheco I, Gerardo R. Aflatoxins biochemistry and molecular biology - biotechnological approaches for control in crops. In: Torres-Pacheco I, editor. Aflatoxins - Detection, Measurement and Control [Internet]. London, UK: InTechOpen; 2011. Available from: http://www.intechopen.com/books/aflatoxins-detection-measurement-and-control/aflatoxins-biochemistry-and-molecular-biology-biotechnological-approaches-for-control-in-crops [Accessed: February 26, 2024]

[23] Guevara-Gonzalez RG. Aflatoxins: Biochemistry and Molecular Biology. Norderstedt, Germany: BoD–Books on Demand; 2011

[24] Bhatnagar D, Ehrlich KC, Cleveland TE. Molecular genetic analysis and regulation of aflatoxin biosynthesis. Applied Microbiology and Biotechnology. 2003;**61**(2):83-93

[25] Price MS, Yu J, Nierman WC, Kim HS, Pritchard B, Jacobus CA, et al. The aflatoxin pathway regulator AflR induces gene transcription inside and outside of the aflatoxin biosynthetic cluster. FEMS Microbiology Letters. 2006;**255**(2):275-279

[26] Bhatnagar-Mathur P, Sunkara S, Bhatnagar-Panwar M, Waliyar F, Sharma KK. Biotechnological advances for combating *aspergillus flavus* and

aflatoxin contamination in crops. Plant Science. 2015;**234**:119-132

[27] Nazhand A, Durazzo A, Lucarini M, Souto EB, Santini A. Characteristics, occurrence, detection and detoxification of aflatoxins in foods and feeds. Food. 2020;**9**(5):644

[28] Yang Y, Li G, Wu D, Liu J, Li X, Luo P, et al. Recent advances on toxicity and determination methods of mycotoxins in foodstuffs. Trends in Food Science & Technology. 2020;**96**:233-252

[29] Alshannaq A, Yu JH. Occurrence, toxicity, and analysis of major mycotoxins in food. International Journal of Environmental Research and Public Health. 2017;**14**(6):632

[30] McMillan A, Renaud JB, Burgess KMN, Orimadegun AE, Akinyinka OO, Allen SJ, et al. Aflatoxin exposure in Nigerian children with severe acute malnutrition. Food and Chemical Toxicology. 2018;**111**:356-362

[31] Kumar P, Mahato DK, Kamle M, Mohanta TK, Kang SG. Aflatoxins: A global concern for food safety, human health and their management. Frontiers in Microbiology [Internet]. 2017;**07**. Available from: http://journal.frontiersin.org/article/10.3389/fmicb.2016.02170/full [Accessed: December 11, 2024]

[32] Sharma S, Gupta D, Sharma YP. Natural incidence of aflatoxins, Ochratoxin a, Patulin and their Co-occurrence in Chilgoza pine nuts marketed in Jammu, India. Proceedings of the National Academy of Sciences, India Section B: Biological Sciences. 2015;**85**(1):45-50

[33] Iqbal SZ, Mehmood Z, Asi MR, Shahid M, Sehar M, Malik N. Co-occurrence of aflatoxins and ochratoxin a in nuts, dry fruits, and nuty products. Journal of Food Safety. 2018;**38**(4):e12462

[34] Adetunji MC, Alika OP, Awa NP, Atanda OO, Mwanza M. Microbiological quality and risk assessment for aflatoxins in groundnuts and roasted cashew nuts meant for human consumption. Journal of Toxicology. 2018;**2018**:1-11

[35] Kamika I, Ngbolua K te N, Tekere M. Occurrence of aflatoxin contamination in maize throughout the supply chain in the Democratic Republic of Congo. Food Control. 2016;**69**:292-296

[36] Kaaya AN, Kyamuhangire W. The effect of storage time and agroecological zone on mould incidence and aflatoxin contamination of maize from traders in Uganda. International Journal of Food Microbiology. 2006;**110**(3):217-223

[37] Mutiga SK, Hoffmann V, Harvey JW, Milgroom MG, Nelson RJ. Assessment of aflatoxin and Fumonisin contamination of maize in Western Kenya. Phytopathology. 2015;**105**(9):1250-1261

[38] Ayar A, Sert D, Çon AH. A study on the occurrence of aflatoxin In raw Milk due to feeds. Journal of Food Safety. 2007;**27**(2):199-207

[39] Gizachew D, Szonyi B, Tegegne A, Hanson J, Grace D. Aflatoxin contamination of milk and dairy feeds in the greater Addis Ababa milk shed, Ethiopia. Food Control. 2016;**59**:773-779

[40] Daou R, Afif C, Joubrane K, Khabbaz LR, Maroun R, Ismail A, et al. Occurrence of aflatoxin M1 in raw, pasteurized, UHT cows' milk, and dairy products in Lebanon. Food Control. 2020;**111**:107055

[41] O'Riordan MJ, Wilkinson MG. A survey of the incidence and level of aflatoxin contamination in a range of

imported spice preparations on the Irish retail market. Food Chemistry. 2008;**107**(4):1429-1435

[42] Ali N, Hashim NH, Shuib NS. Natural occurrence of aflatoxins and ochratoxin A in processed spices marketed in Malaysia. Food Additives & Contaminants: Part A. 2015;**32**(4):518-532

[43] Ozbey F, Kabak B. Natural co-occurrence of aflatoxins and ochratoxin a in spices. Food Control. 2012;**28**(2):354-361

[44] Armorini S, Altafini A, Zaghini A, Roncada P. Occurrence of aflatoxin B1 in conventional and organic flour in Italy and the role of sampling. Food Control. 2015;**50**:858-863

[45] Kara GN, Ozbey F, Kabak B. Co-occurrence of aflatoxins and ochratoxin a in cereal flours commercialised in Turkey. Food Control. 2015;**54**:275-281

[46] Taheri N, Semnani S, Roshandel G, Namjoo M, Keshavarzian H, Chogan A, et al. Aflatoxin contamination in wheat flour samples from Golestan Province, northeast of Iran. Iranian Journal of Public Health. 2012;**41**(9):42-47

[47] Klich MA. Environmental and developmental factors influencing aflatoxin production by *aspergillus flavus* and *aspergillus parasiticus*. Mycoscience. 2007;**48**(2):71-80

[48] Kumar A, Pathak H, Bhadauria S, Sudan J. Aflatoxin contamination in food crops: Causes, detection, and management: A review. Food Production, Processing and Nutrition. 2021;**3**(1):17

[49] Wu F. Global impacts of aflatoxin in maize: Trade and human health. World Mycotoxin Journal. 2015;**8**(2):137-142

[50] Mitchell NJ, Bowers E, Hurburgh C, Wu F. Potential economic losses to the US corn industry from aflatoxin contamination. Food Additives & Contaminants: Part A. 2016;**33**(3):540-550

[51] Dewey KG, Adu-Afarwuah S. Systematic review of the efficacy and effectiveness of complementary feeding interventions in developing countries. Maternal & Child Nutrition. 2008;**4**(s1):24-85

[52] U.S. Department of Health and Human Services, Food and Drug Administration, Center for Food Safety, Applied Nutrition, Office of Regulatory Affairs. Compliance Policy Guide Sec. 555.400 Aflatoxins in Human Food: Guidance for FDA Staff. FDA; 2021. p. 5

[53] The Commission of The European Communitie. Commission Regulation (EC) No 1881/2006 Setting Maximum Levels for Certain Contaminants in Foodstuffs. EC regulation; 2006. p. 35

[54] Marin DE, Taranu I. Overview on aflatoxins and oxidative stress. Toxin Reviews. 2012;**31**(3-4):32-43

[55] Li C, Liu X, Wu J, Ji X, Xu Q. Research progress in toxicological effects and mechanism of aflatoxin B_1 toxin. PeerJ. 2022;**10**:e13850

[56] Qiang M. In: Pohjanvirta R, editor. The AH Receptor in Biology and Toxicology [Internet]. 1st ed. New Jersey, USA: Wiley; 2011. DOI: 10.1002/9781118140574 [Accessed: December 1, 2024]

[57] Arenas-Huertero F, Zaragoza-Ojeda M, Sánchez-Alarcón J, Milić M, Šegvić Klarić M, Montiel-González JM, et al. Involvement of Ahr pathway in toxicity of aflatoxins and other mycotoxins. Frontiers in Microbiology. 2019;**10**:2347

[58] Wang Z, Snyder M, Kenison JE, Yang K, Lara B, Lydell E, et al. How the AHR became important in cancer: The role of chronically active AHR in cancer aggression. International Journal of Molecular Sciences. 2020;**22**(1):387

[59] Wang Z, Monti S, Sherr DH. The diverse and important contributions of the AHR to cancer and cancer immunity. Current Opinion in Toxicology. 2017;**2**:93-102

[60] Pot C. Aryl hydrocarbon receptor controls regulatory CD4+T cell function. Hochdorf, Switzerland: Swiss Medical Weekly [Internet]; 2012. Available from: https://smw.ch/index.php/smw/article/view/1494 [Accessed: December 1, 2024]

[61] Benkerroum N. Chronic and acute toxicities of aflatoxins: Mechanisms of action. International Journal of Environmental Research and Public Health. 2020;**17**(2):423

[62] Lin YC, Li L, Makarova AV, Burgers PM, Stone MP, Lloyd RS. Error-prone replication bypass of the primary aflatoxin B1 DNA adduct, AFB1-N7-Gua. Journal of Biological Chemistry. 2014;**289**(26):18497-18506

[63] Hafner A, Bulyk ML, Jambhekar A, Lahav G. The multiple mechanisms that regulate p53 activity and cell fate. Nature Reviews. Molecular Cell Biology. 2019;**20**(4):199-210

[64] Long XD, Deng Y, Huang XY, Yao JG, Su QY, Wu XM, et al. Molecular mechanisms of hepatocellular carcinoma related to aflatoxins: An update. In: Rodrigo L, editor. Liver Research and Clinical Management [Internet]. London, UK: InTechOpen; 2018. Available from: http://www.intechopen.com/books/liver-research-and-clinical-management/molecular-mechanisms-of-hepatocellular-carcinoma-related-to-aflatoxins-an-update [Accessed: July 9, 2024]

[65] Moudgil V, Redhu D, Dhanda S, Singh J. A review of molecular mechanisms in the development of hepatocellular carcinoma by aflatoxin and hepatitis B and C viruses. Journal of Environmental Pathology, Toxicology and Oncology. 2013;**32**(2):165-175

[66] Mizrak D, Engin B, Onder FO, Yener B, Bektas M, Biyikli Z, et al. Aflatoxin exposure in viral hepatitis patients in Turkey. The Turkish Journal of Gastroenterology. 2009;**20**(3):192-197

[67] Ruan H, Lu Q, Wu J, Qin J, Sui M, Sun X, et al. Hepatotoxicity of food-borne mycotoxins: Molecular mechanism, anti-hepatotoxic medicines and target prediction. Critical Reviews in Food Science and Nutrition. 2022;**62**(9):2281-2308

[68] Fan T, Xie Y, Ma W. Research progress on the protection and detoxification of phytochemicals against aflatoxin B1-induced liver toxicity. Toxicon. 2021;**195**:58-68

[69] Kipkoech G, Jepkorir M, Kamau S, Wanyoko A, Kibunja S, Amozi Jeremiah R, et al. Immunomodulatory effects of aflatoxin B1 (AFB1) and the use of natural products to ameliorate its immunotoxic effects: A review. Open Research Africa. 2023;**6**:22

[70] He XN, Zeng ZZ, Wu P, Jiang WD, Liu Y, Jiang J, et al. Dietary aflatoxin B1 attenuates immune function of immune organs in grass carp (*Ctenopharyngodon idella*) by modulating NF-κB and the TOR signaling pathway. Frontiers in Immunology [Internet]. 2022;**13**:1027064. Available from: https://www.frontiersin.org/articles/10.3389/fimmu.2022.1027064/full [Accessed: January 3, 2025]

[71] Blevins HM, Xu Y, Biby S, Zhang S. The NLRP3 Inflammasome pathway: A review of mechanisms and inhibitors for the treatment of inflammatory diseases. Frontiers in Aging Neuroscience [Internet]. 2022;**14**:879021. Available from: https://www.frontiersin.org/articles/10.3389/fnagi.2022.879021/full

[72] Fan W, Lv Y, Ren S, Shao M, Shen T, Huang K, et al. Zearalenone (ZEA)-induced intestinal inflammation is mediated by the NLRP3 inflammasome. Chemosphere [Internet]. 2018;**190**:272-279. Available from: https://linkinghub.elsevier.com/retrieve/pii/S0045653517315679

[73] Zha A, Cui Z, Qi M, Liao S, Chen L, Liao P, et al. Dietary baicalin zinc supplementation alleviates oxidative stress and enhances nutrition absorption in deoxynivalenol challenged pigs. Current Drug Metabolism [Internet]. 2020;**21**(8):614-625. Available from: https://www.eurekaselect.com/179871/article

[74] Taranu I, Hermenean A, Bulgaru C, Pistol GC, Ciceu A, Grosu IA, et al. Diet containing grape seed meal by-product counteracts AFB1 toxicity in liver of pig after weaning. Ecotoxicology and Environmental Safety [Internet]. 2020;**203**:110899. Available from: https://linkinghub.elsevier.com/retrieve/pii/S0147651320307387

[75] He Q, Suzuki H, Sharma N, Sharma RP. Ceramide synthase inhibition by Fumonisin B1 treatment activates sphingolipid-metabolizing systems in mouse liver. Toxicological Sciences [Internet]. 2006;**94**(2):388-397. DOI: 10.1093/toxsci/kfl102

[76] Sharma RP, He Q, Johnson VJ. Deletion of IFN- γ reduces Fumonisin-induced hepatotoxicity in mice via alterations in inflammatory cytokines and apoptotic factors. Journal of Interferon & Cytokine Research [Internet]. 2003;**23**(1):13-23. DOI: 10.1089/10799900360520414

[77] Afonina IS, Zhong Z, Karin M, Beyaert R. Limiting inflammation—The negative regulation of NF-κB and the NLRP3 inflammasome. Nature Immunology [Internet]. 2017;**18**(8):861-869. Available from: https://www.nature.com/articles/ni.3772

[78] Zhang J, Su D, Liu Q, Yuan Q, Ouyang Z, Wei Y, et al. Gasdermin D-mediated microglial pyroptosis exacerbates neurotoxicity of aflatoxins B1 and M1 in mouse primary microglia and neuronal cultures. Neurotoxicology [Internet]. 2022;**91**:305-320. Available from: https://linkinghub.elsevier.com/retrieve/pii/S0161813X22000948

[79] Swanson KV, Deng M, Ting JPY. The NLRP3 inflammasome: Molecular activation and regulation to therapeutics. Nature Reviews. Immunology [Internet]. 2019;**19**(8):477-489. Available from: https://www.nature.com/articles/s41577-019-0165-0

[80] Dai C, Tian E, Li H, Gupta SD, Hao Z, Wang Z, et al. Molecular mechanisms of aflatoxin neurotoxicity and potential neuroprotective agents. Food Science and Human Wellness [Internet]. 2024;**13**(5):2445-2455. Available from: https://www.sciopen.com/article/10.26599/FSHW.2022.9250201

Chapter 3

Biological Strategies for Aflatoxin Mitigation in Food and Feed Chains in a Changing World

María Silvina Alaniz-Zanon, Marianela Bossa, María Laura Chiotta and Sofía Noemí Chulze

Abstract

Aflatoxins (AFs) are secondary metabolites produced by *Aspergillus* section *Flavi*, mainly *Aspergillus flavus* and *Aspergillus parasiticus.* These species may infect food and feed along entire agri-food chains, synthesizing the toxin when environmental conditions are favorable. The scenario of climate change that the world will have to face in the next decades is expected to increase the levels of AF contamination in cereals, nuts, spices, and legumes, among other important crops around the world. This situation will have a great impact on human and animal health, as well as economic losses due to the rejection of contaminated products during commercialization. Several mitigation strategies have been implemented to counteract this problem. Some of them are intended to prevent AF synthesis, while others are designed to decontaminate the pre-formed toxin. In addition, several pre- and post-harvest strategies have shown effectivity. Besides physical and chemical tools, biological control based on different microorganisms and the use of enzymes have been proposed as promissory approaches to mitigate the risk of AF contamination. In this chapter, detailed information about two developments is presented: biocontrol based on prevention by a non-toxigenic *A. flavus* strain and the use of fungal laccases to decontaminate AFs. The integration of these tools will enhance the quality of food and feed, contributing to food safety in agri-food chains.

Keywords: aflatoxins, food and feed chains, mitigation strategies, climate change, biocontrol, enzymes

1. Introduction

This chapter aims to provide a compilation of existing and updated information on aflatoxin (AFs) contamination in agriculturally important crops around the world, as well as the most promising strategies to mitigate this contamination in the context of climate change, thus contributing to food security and preserving human and animal health.

Aflatoxins (AFs), harmful metabolites synthesized by *Aspergillus* section *Flavi,* mainly *A. flavus* and *A. parasiticus*, among others, are naturally occurring pollutants in food and feed chains. While AFs have posed an issue throughout history, they have only been recognized as major contaminants in agriculture since the 1960s, after an outbreak in turkeys from England during 1960 [1]. Since then, many efforts have been done to control, reduce, and/or eliminate AFs in the production chains. Among the several developed strategies, chemical, physical, and biological techniques have been described. These strategies have their limitations in terms of efficiency, cost, and potential effects on food quality, highlighting the need for a multifaceted approach to effectively prevent contamination [2].

Aflatoxins are synthesized during hydric and thermic stresses. In this context, the scenario of climate change predicted for next decades would enhance not only the incidence and severity of agricultural crop diseases but also mycotoxin accumulation. Over the next 10–25 years, an increase in temperature of 2–5°C, elevated CO_2 levels (current: 400 ppm currently vs. future: 1000 ppm), and cycles of severe drought alternating with periods of intense moisture are expected [3]. This situation makes it even more critical to develop and implement effective strategies for controlling mycotoxin levels.

Throughout this chapter, information about the diversity of crops affected by toxigenic *Aspergillus* section *Flavi* and AFs is provided. During both pre- and post-harvest stages, fungal infection and mycotoxin contamination may occur, and mycotoxin levels may increase during handling and storage. In this sense, a general description of the first steps regarding the management of AFs is addressed. In addition, two of the most promising biological tools to date for mitigation of AF contamination are described in this chapter: (1) control based on the use of biocontrol agents during pre-harvest stage, and (2) a post-harvest tool based on fungal enzymes for the decontamination of AFs.

2. Aflatoxins in economically important crops

The Food and Agriculture Organization of the United Nations (FAO) estimates that 45 countries around the world require external support for food. Conflicts and wars caused by mainly religious and political reasons in different regions are contributing to dangerously high levels of severe acute food insecurity, while widespread drought conditions are anticipated to worsen this situation [4]. Additionally, plant diseases and pests contribute to as much as 40% of global food production losses, resulting in an annual estimated global loss of 40 billion dollars, both directly and indirectly [5]. According to FAO, around 25% of the world's food crops are vulnerable to infection by plant pathogenic fungi and contamination by mycotoxins [6].

Foods considered most susceptible to fungal contamination with the subsequent production of AFs typically include maize, peanuts, pistachios, walnuts and almonds, rice, figs, melon, and seeds, among others, in both producing and exporting countries worldwide [1, 7]. Aflatoxins have also been found in oilseeds such as sunflower and soybeans; in unrefined vegetable oils; in spices like paprika, chili, and pepper; in dried fruits like dried figs and raisins; in coffee and cocoa, and in other cereals and their derived products [8]. Considering the multiplicity of substrates that can be contaminated with AFs, the highly variable contamination levels, and the wide range of factors that determine the risks associated with this contamination, it is difficult to provide a generalized summary. Therefore, only a few examples will be presented below.

Cereal grains are typically consumed either raw or cooked or transformed into processed items like flour, semolina, bread, and cookies. Additionally, cereal crops and their sub-products are commonly used as feed for livestock and poultry, which in turn serve as inputs to produce dairy, poultry, and meat products for human consumption. Some of those cereals that have been reported with AF contamination are rice, maize, barley, sorghum, and wheat, among others.

Rice is a vital staple food worldwide, ranking third in global consumption after wheat. It accounts for 27% of the world's energy intake and provides 20% of dietary protein in developing nations [9]. Various authors have reported AF contamination levels higher than the established limits (5 and 10 μg/kg for AFB_1 and total AFs, respectively) in several countries [10, 11].

Maize is the second-most cultivated crop worldwide after rice, and AF outbreaks in this substrate are a significant public health concern, particularly in sub-Saharan Africa, where environmental conditions and agricultural practices contribute to contamination. In 1974, an aflatoxicosis outbreak causing hepatitis was reported in India, producing the death of 106 people and also affecting dogs. After that, more outbreaks were reported in humans (both adults and children) and chickens in this country [12, 13]. In 2004, one of the most significant aflatoxicosis outbreaks, involving maize, took place in rural Kenya, leading to 317 cases and 125 deaths [14]. Tanzania and Southern and Eastern Europe have also suffered AF consequences associated to contaminated maize or sub-products [15, 16]. An interesting and worrying case occurred in 2013, when significant levels of AFM_1 (product of the biotransformation of AFB_1 in certain animals that have consumed contaminated feed) were detected in milk tanks in the Netherlands and Germany, as a consequence of which farmers had accidentally fed cows with maize contaminated with AFs. During the maize growing season of 2012, high AF concentrations were found in Serbia, Bulgaria, Romania, Hungary, Ukraine, Spain, Italy, Greece, and Poland [17].

Soil is the primary source of AF-producing fungi, and since peanut fruits grow underground, their pods come into direct contact with these fungal populations. In 2001, peanut samples harvested in Argentina showed high levels of total AFs [18]. A survey carried out in Nigeria reported that 90% of the analyzed samples contained AFB_1 above the allowed limits [19]. Pistachio commercialization is an important market in several countries. In some pistachio batches, AF levels above the maximum established limits were detected [7]. A similar situation has been observed for Brazil nuts [20]. Although peanuts and pistachios are the most frequent reported nuts with AF contamination, others such as hazelnuts and almonds are also of great concern worldwide [21].

A survey developed in chickpeas in Pakistan revealed that 62% of the samples were contaminated with AFB_1 [22]. Other legumes like lentils have also been reported with AF contamination [23]. However, considering the occurrence of *A. flavus* in this substrate and the changing climate conditions, further studies would be necessary.

In recent decades, the incidence of mycotoxicosis in humans has risen due to the consumption of food contaminated with one or more mycotoxins, including AFs. In this sense, it is relevant to focus the efforts on two main stages: detection and management. The next sections will describe some of the most popular and promissory strategies, with focus on the management tools.

3. Aflatoxin control approaches

Over the years, AFs have led to the loss of human and animal lives, and if not so far, they have driven important economic losses. Thus, the history of AF mitigation strategies has evolved significantly. Management approaches for these mycotoxins may be focused on different stages of the production processes: at field stage (pre-harvest), during storage, and during processing (post-harvest), as mycotoxins can be produced throughout the whole agri-food chain (**Figure 1**). Environmental factors, particularly water availability and temperature, which influence the infection by toxigenic fungi and consequently the contamination levels of these toxins, are critical aspects to consider [24, 25].

Several methods based on detection tools have been improved over time, including chromatographic and molecular techniques, which are crucial for early identification of AF contamination [26]. However, sampling continues to be a critical point since there is significant variability in AF distribution across a batch of bulk kernels [27]. Complimentarily, the regulation of public and health policies is mandatory in AF mitigation [28]. In this sense, many countries have established maximum allowed limits for the commercialization of raw materials and products intended for human and animal feed.

Good agricultural practices were one of the first efficient management methods used by farmers [29]. Some of them include the use of drought-tolerant varieties, timely harvesting before physiological maturity, sorting to remove damaged ears and

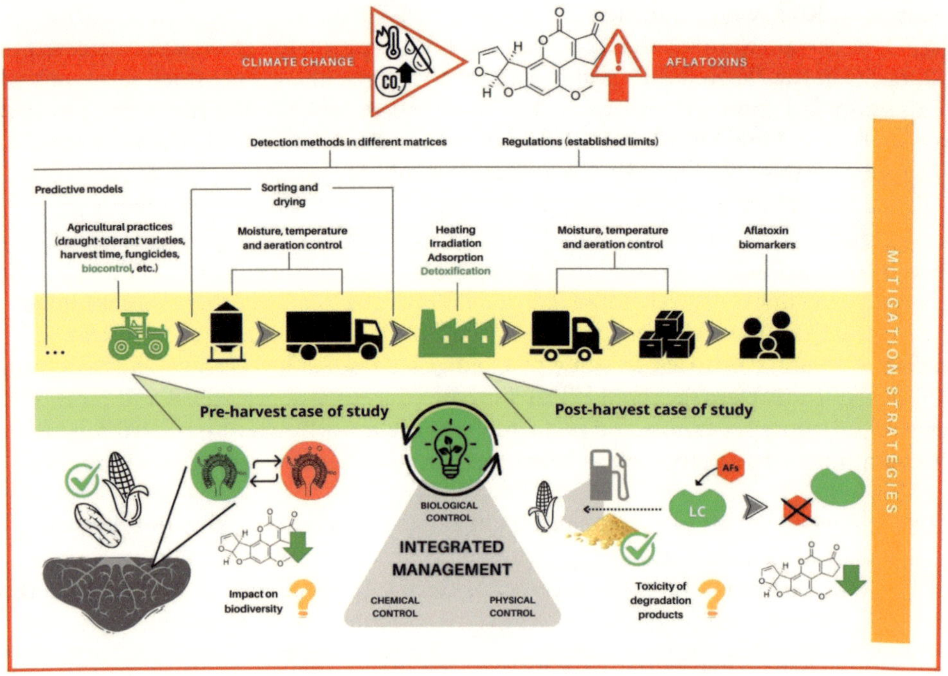

Figure 1.
Strategies to mitigate AFs in agri-food chains under a climate-change scenario. Climate change will favor an increase in aflatoxin (AFs) contamination of food and feed along the entire agri-food chains. Several tools have been proved to mitigate aflatoxins along productive chains. In a context of an integrated management of AF contamination, two complementary biological control tools have been developed for pre- and post-harvest stages, among other chemical and physical tools. At pre-harvest, the application of a biocontrol agent based on a non-toxigenic Aspergillus flavus *strain (indicated with an* Aspergillus *head in a green circle) that competes with native toxigenic strains (indicated with an* Aspergillus *head in a red circle) is able to prevent AF accumulation in maize and peanut kernels. Another biological supplementary strategy is the use of fungal laccases to decontaminate AFs during bioethanol production from maize, where co-products are intended for animal feed. Both technologies contribute to food safety. However, some aspects, such as the environmental impact and the toxicity of the degradation products, as well as several developments to control AFs, need to be deeply studied.*

those having poor husk covering, drying properly to specific percentages of moisture content, and storage in suitable conditions to keep the crop clean and under conditions with minimally proper aeration or ideally under hermetic conditions [30].

Incorporating resistant crop varieties, such as sorghum, into animal feed can lower AF levels in dairy products [31]. Regarding maize, plant breeding and varietal selection have been used to develop disease-resistant varieties [32]. Even this approach has led to the identification of several maize lines that exhibit resistance to *A. flavus* invasion, but up to now, no commercial varieties are available. In peanuts, an effectiveness of up to 100% was observed using resistant genotypes [33]. Also, in rice, the use of specific varieties of this crop had a significant impact in AF accumulation [34]. However, these resistant varieties face several limitations that hinder their effectiveness. These limitations include the complexity of genetic resistance, environmental influences, and the incomplete protection offered by current resistant varieties.

The first physical strategy to mitigate AFs involved manual visual sorting, which has been widely recognized for its effectiveness, particularly in peanuts. Studies indicate that this method can effectively reduce AF content by a significant percentage (56-99% in combination with other methods), making it a practical approach in low-income countries, despite being tedious and not eliminating all contaminated kernels [35, 36]. Other physical methods include heating above 160°C [37], irradiation [38], and adsorption by different kinds of adsorbents, nanoparticles, nanocomposites, and magnetic-activated carbon, which have been demonstrated as suitable agents for AFB_1 decontamination in poultry feed and vegetable oils [39].

Regarding chemical strategies, the use of fungicides has been a primary method for controlling aflatoxigenic fungi [40]. Over time, various chemical approaches have evolved, including the development of natural-based compounds, bioactive agents, synthetic antioxidants, nanoparticles, and microencapsulated and encapsulated formulations with variable efficiency and limitations such as application methodologies [41, 42].

While effective, these physical and chemical methods may not fully eliminate AFs, highlighting the need for further research into more comprehensive strategies for AF management in food safety, such as biological control at pre- and post-harvest stages.

4. Pre-harvest biocontrol strategies

Three intervention levels have been described to reduce AF accumulation in food and feed chains: prevention, decontamination, and detoxification [39]. Generally, pre-harvest strategies are intended to prevent AF synthesis through different mechanisms. Considering the potential shift in AF occurrence patterns in food and feed because of climate change, this matter may need anticipatory actions [43]. In this context, several predictive models based on statistical tools have been proposed for different crops such as maize, pistachio, and peanuts. Other models consider machine learning approaches [44, 45]. However, each of these models are limited to a particular crop, region, climatic characteristics, and agricultural practices.

On the contrary, biocontrol has emerged as a prominent and global strategy for managing AF contamination. Various potential biocontrol agents based on microorganisms with different mechanisms of action have been proved (**Figure 2**) [46]. For instance, *Trichoderma* species have been identified as effective biological control agents, utilizing mechanisms such as antibiosis and mycoparasitism to suppress aflatoxigenic fungi [47].

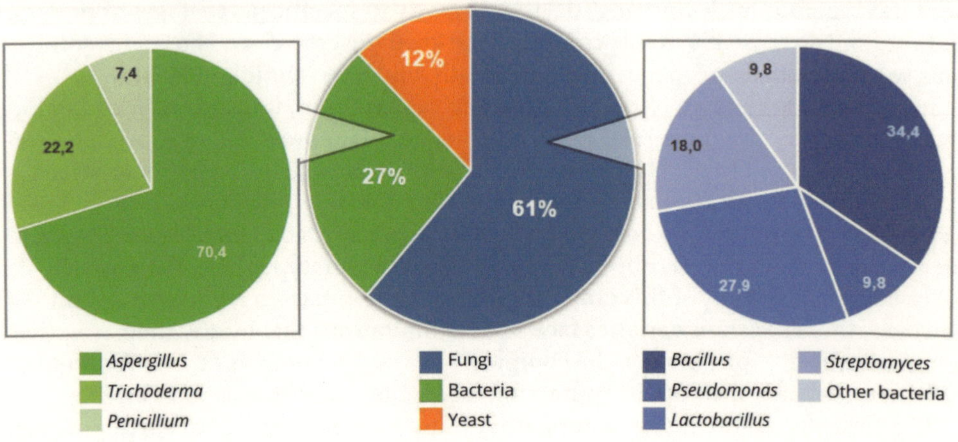

Figure 2.
Microorganisms evaluated as potential biological control agents to reduce aflatoxin accumulation in crops. Adapted from Krska et al. [46].

To date, the widely researched approach that has demonstrated the greatest effectiveness among biological control agents to mitigate AFs involves the use of non-aflatoxigenic strains of *Aspergillus flavus* or *A. parasiticus* to inhibit AF-producing strains. This approach has been validated in various agricultural settings including peanuts, cotton, and maize, and some of them are currently commercially available [48].

When developing a bio-input, many aspects must be considered in addition to effectiveness. Several inoculum preparation methods have been described using different matrices or directly attaching dried conidia (previously grown on culture media) to a carrier. In most of the cases, the bio-input has been applied as a solid formulation. Some matrices have included alginate-based formulations [49] and the use of cereal kernels such as wheat [50], barley [51], and long-grain rice [52, 53]. Other options include the use of bioplastics [51, 54], water-dispersible granules containing tapioca starch [55], the recycling of bioplastic pellets [56], and the development of a biopolymer made from maize starch.

The inoculum rate is another important issue since it may be related with the facility of application as well as the investment that the producer must make to acquire the product. Additionally, application rates may vary depending on the specific characteristics of the crop and the formulation [53, 57–59]. Furthermore, depending on the life cycle of *Aspergillus* in the crop, different application methods have been evaluated considering the phenology of each crop, artificial or natural irrigation, one or more applications, and frequent cultural practices, among other factors [59, 60].

In general, the development of bio-inputs is driven by a range of technological innovations combined with the use of cost-effective and available substrates to lower production investments. Solid-state fermentation (SSF) offers several advantages regarding technological, economic, environmental, and biological factors. Although submerged fermentation provides greater consistency in the system, a broader range of applications, and better regulation of environmental conditions, SSF remains the preferred method for agricultural bio-input production due to its cost-effectiveness, ease of implementation, and simplicity in maintenance by farmers. Evaluating productivity is essential for the large-scale production and worldwide use of bio-inputs. Both the parameters of the production process and the composition of the substrate influence the kinetics of microbial metabolism. As a result, selecting the appropriate microbial strain is critical to optimizing either biomass or the production of desired metabolites. Several recent studies have aimed to develop suitable models for scaling up SSF. Many of these works focus on the economic aspects of the process, while a significant portion concentrates on optimizing factors like microbial growth and substrate behavior to improve production [61].

4.1 Environmental impact of bio-inputs and regulatory considerations

Added to the global concern about AF contamination, it has been studied that soil biodiversity is decreasing daily due to various factors, including climate change; intensive cropping; the abuse of agrochemicals; soil, air, and water pollution, and so on [62]. Since microorganisms play an important role in crop health and productivity, it is important to implement AF control strategies that do not threaten microorganism biodiversity. It is known that the introduction of microorganisms into the ecosystem can influence, at least temporarily, not only the native microbial communities but also the efficiency of biocontrol [63, 64]. In this context, it is relevant to use native strains as biocontrol agents, minimizing the environmental impact. Therefore, although these strategies have shown promise, challenges remain, and continuous innovation and adaptation of mitigation strategies are essential to ensure food safety and public health.

The regulatory considerations for bio-inputs regarding environmental impacts are crucial for ensuring sustainable agricultural practices. There is a pressing need for comprehensive regulations that address their production, use, and environmental effects [65]. Also, in many countries, there is a requirement of several assessments, including evaluating gene flow, effects on non-target organisms, and biodiversity impacts. However, these analyses involve subjective judgments about acceptable risks, complicating the regulatory process. Additionally, post-commercialization monitoring is essential to assess long-term impacts, yet it presents challenges in measurement and verification. Therefore, while bio-inputs offer a sustainable alternative to harmful pesticides, the lack of robust regulatory frameworks may hinder their potential benefits. Addressing these gaps is essential for balancing agricultural productivity with environmental protection [66].

4.2 *Aspergillus flavus* as a biocontrol agent for aflatoxin management in maize and peanuts: Case of study

Maize and peanuts are crops of great importance worldwide and particularly for Argentina [67]. Although, in general, climatic conditions do not typically favor AF contamination at the pre-harvest stage, in some seasons and under conditions of high temperatures and low precipitation, concerning levels of these mycotoxins have been detected [58, 68]. Our research group has developed a strategy to prevent AF accumulation in grains, contributing to food safety (**Figure 1**).

Aspergillus flavus is the predominant species within section *Flavi* both in soil and in peanuts harvested in Córdoba province, Argentina. In an initial study, strains with potential use as biocontrol agents were identified. That is, strains not producing either AFs or another mycotoxin called cyclopiazonic acid (CPA) [18, 69]. Additionally, morphological and genetic studies were conducted in order to guarantee a reduced likelihood of genetic exchange with toxigenic strains and to ensure a low probability of sexual reproduction, preventing the production of AFs in their progeny [69, 70]. Chiotta et al. [71] performed a field trial on peanut crops to evaluate the effect of different inoculum rates of a biocontrol strain on AF accumulation in peanuts, with promising results.

Subsequently, Alaniz Zanon [72] evaluated and characterized new populations of *Aspergillus* section *Flavi* isolated from the core peanut-growing region of Argentina. In this work, several analyses were included: morphological parameters, toxigenic profile, molecular analysis based on markers from the AFs and CPA gene clusters, and genetic studies. Moreover, the competitive ability of some pre-selected strains was evaluated under *in situ* assays on peanut and maize kernels, since maize is a key crop in rotation with peanuts in this agricultural region. Bio-formulates based on one or more non-aflatoxigenic strains were studied under field trials in two different agricultural regions to evaluate which one had the best performance [53, 58].

From this research, strains with relevant characteristics were selected for use as biocontrol agents. They demonstrated high competitiveness in peanuts, significantly reducing AF synthesis by a highly aflatoxigenic strain co-inoculated in the *in situ* competition assays. These strains were effective in maize kernels under laboratory conditions. In the field trials on peanuts, reductions in AF contamination ranged from 75 to 86%. The safety of the bioformulation was confirmed in animal assays, and stability during storage of the bio-input under controlled temperature conditions was demonstrated [72].

The research was then extended to maize crops [73]. New *Aspergillus* section *Flavi* strains were isolated, and they were characterized with the same criteria. Many of them were good candidates as biocontrol agents. For a pre-selection, *in situ* competition assays were conducted on maize kernels. Two strains (*A. flavus* AFCHG2 and ARG5-30) were evaluated at the field stage, both individually and in a mixed formulation, analyzing their residual effect on kernels stored under different conditions. At the field stage, all the tested formulations were able to displace native toxigenic strains, thus reducing AF contamination. In Argentina and other countries, silo-bag technology has become a predominant method for the storage of dry kernels and forage. In this research, we demonstrated that the field application of biocontrol agents is an effective tool for reducing the risk of AF accumulation in maize kernels stored in hermetic silo-bags for 3 and 6 months [24].

Simultaneously, with the aim to replace rice (that serves as food and feed), a macroporous biopolymer based on maize starch was developed as substrate and carrier for the biocontrol agent. This biopolymer is biodegradable and has good mechanical properties and a significant macroporosity that allows the biocontrol agent to grow within the solid matrix (patent request submitted to the Instituto Nacional de la Propiedad Industrial, Argentina, web reference number 1682840). In additional field trials, growth of bioformulates of *A. flavus* AFCHG2 on long-grain rice and on the biopolymer was evaluated, with no significant differences in the effectiveness on reducing AFs.

In preliminary field studies recently conducted on maize, it was demonstrated that the application of bioformulations based on *A. flavus* strains AFCHG2 and ARG5-30 did not have an environmental impact on soil fungal diversity. In addition, it was confirmed that both biocontrol strains (AFCHG2 and ARG5-30) are effective in controlling AFB_1 contamination under simulated climatic conditions [74]. Additional research is being conducted to extend this knowledge.

5. Post-harvest biocontrol strategies

When pre-harvest strategies are not efficient enough, are not available, or are impracticable, post-harvest tools are necessary to complement, correct, or apply mitigation actions. Some post-harvest tools are intended to prevent AF accumulation, but most of them are focused on AF elimination, biotransformation, decontamination, and detoxification.

The main strategies for post-harvest mycotoxin mitigation are based on controlling moisture, water activity of the grains, and temperature during storage and transportation [75]. Additionally, in food processing, several physical and chemical decontamination treatments can be used to reduce mycotoxin levels, such as sorting and sieving, washing, milling, thermal treatment, grain irradiation, and the use of adsorbents, as previously mentioned. Chemical methods such as ammoniation, treatment with different acids, alkaline hydrolysis, peroxidation, and the use of bisulfites are available to reduce mycotoxins. Nevertheless, their application in food and feed is limited due to potential toxicity, low effectiveness, high costs, and adverse effects on the quality of raw materials [76]. Recently, other technologies based on physical methods have been described, such as fluorescence sorting of grains [39, 77], pulsed electric fields for liquid matrices, and pulsed ultrasonic radiation. However, some of these methods cause significant structural changes and inactivation of proteins and enzymes in the matrix [78]. Cold plasma treatment of food has shown effectiveness (100% decontamination in less than 120 seconds) in controlling fungi and their toxins while preserving the characteristics of the matrix [79]. Regarding chemical methods, nanoparticles, nanocomposites, magnetic activated carbon, and ozone have shown promising although variable results (25-100% AF reduction) [80].

In the post-harvest stage, biological methods are based on the use of microorganisms and/or their enzymes to metabolize, destroy, or deactivate toxins, transforming them into stable, less toxic, and even harmless compounds [81]. The evaluation of the toxicity and safety of degradation products of AFs is of utmost importance, as they may pose a risk equal to or greater than that of the original compounds, thus threatening both human and animal health.

A wide variety of microorganisms and their enzymes have been capable of degrading AFs, such as *Pseudomonas*, *Rhodococcus*, *Streptomyces*, and *Bacillus*, as well as *Saccharomyces cerevisiae*. The mechanisms of AF degradation are very diverse, including adsorption, enzymatic degradation, and inhibition of mycotoxin synthesis. Some non-toxigenic strains of *Aspergillus niger* used in the food industry and producers of a large enzymatic battery have also demonstrated the ability to degrade AFB_1 (82-97% degradation) [82]. Regarding mycotoxin degradation by enzymes, several of them have been reported as able to degrade one or more mycotoxins. Specifically for the degradation of AFB_1, different metabolic pathways have been identified, and depending on the enzyme, various and different degradation products are generated [83]. These enzymes include lactonases, oxidoreductases, and others synthetized by some species of *Pantoea* and *Pseudomonas.* Lactonases are produced by species of the *Bacillus* genus, such as *B. megaterium*. On the other hand, the main oxidoreductases studied in AF degradation are oxidases, reductases, peroxidases, and laccases [81].

The AF oxidase enzyme produced by *Armillariella tabescens* was the first enzyme discovered capable of completely degrading this mycotoxin [84]. Meanwhile, AFB_1-degrading reductases are mainly produced by various *Mycobacteria* [85] and *Bacillus subtilis* [86]. Some enzymes of this type have achieved significant reductions of AFB_1 in pistachios [86].

Laccases are multicopper oxidase enzymes that are synthesized by fungi belonging to the phylum Basidiomycota and by other organisms such as plants, bacteria, and insects [87]. In particular, laccases from white-rot fungi stand out for their high redox potential, which makes them applicable in several industries such as paper, textiles, bioremediation, food, and organic synthesis.

The main oxidase enzymes include lignin peroxidase (LiP), manganese peroxidase (MnP), versatile peroxidases, and dye-decolorizing peroxidase (DyP) [87]. Several researchers have identified MnPs as enzymes capable of degrading AFB_1 (up to 94%) [88]. Regarding DyP enzymes, many researchers have expressed these enzymes from fungal and/or bacterial strains in *Escherichia coli*, achieving significant reductions of AFB_1 (up to 96%) [89, 90].

Laccases have been the subject of study for their ability to degrade various mycotoxins, primarily AFB_1. One of the first studies was conducted by Alberts et al. [91]. They evaluated the AFB_1 degradation by a purified laccase from *Trametes versicolor* (1 U/ml), achieving an 87% decontamination. Other studies evaluated purified and unpurified laccases from *P. pulmonaris* and *P. ostreatus*, respectively, and observed 23-76% of reduction in AFB_1 levels [91, 92]. Additionally, it has been shown that the type of substrates targeted by fungal laccases can be expanded through the use of redox mediators, thereby improving the efficiency of their oxidation [93]. In this sense, there are reports that demonstrate the enhancement of the redox potential, showing higher degradation rates of AFB_1 when using acetosyringone [94].

5.1 Fungal laccases for aflatoxin decontamination in the bioethanol production process: Case of study

In Argentina and other parts of the world, co-products from the bioethanol industry, obtained from maize, are used for animal feed either directly or for the preparation of feedstuff [95, 96]. Several studies have shown the presence of AFs in these co-products, which poses a threat to food safety, both for animals and indirectly for humans [97]. This issue is primarily because AF levels concentrate during the production process, reaching up to three times the initial concentration of AFs in maize kernels [98–100]. It is worth mentioning that currently only good agricultural practices are implemented, but no other specific strategy is used to prevent the synthesis of aflatoxins in the pre-harvest stages, such as the use of biocontrol agents. In this context, there is a need to develop a strategy that complements preventive strategies at the field stage, such as the implementation of biological control with a non-toxigenic *A. flavus* strain. Furthermore, the goal for this technology is to reduce AF levels generating innocuous and safe products for animal consumption while being environmentally friendly (**Figure 1**).

Recently, our research group collected and isolated species within the phylum Basidiomycota, including *Funalia trogii, Phellinus tuberculosus, Pleurotus ostreatus, Pycnoporus sanguineus,* and *Trametes gallica*, which showed laccase activity. Strains belonging to the *Trametes gallica* species exhibited the highest specific and enzymatic activities during the periods evaluated. Different laccase isoenzymes were detected among species, but no differences were observed among strains within the same species [101]. Based on these findings, the next step involved decontamination assays to evaluate the effectiveness of these laccase-producing strains in reducing AFs.

Fungal extracts containing laccases were prepared for *in vitro* studies both in buffer and in maize steep liquor in order to evaluate AFB_1 decontamination by these extracts. In these assays, the AFB_1 degradation ability of previous fungal strains was tested in the presence and absence of vanillic acid as a redox mediator. The most effective strain in decontaminating AFB_1 was *T. gallica* B7-IMICO-RC, which was able to reduce this mycotoxin by 87% in the presence of 1 mM vanillic acid and at a laccase enzymatic activity of 20 U/ml. This strain was also effective in degrading the mycotoxin in the absence of the redox mediator, achieving a 66% reduction at the same enzymatic activity, and confirming the enhancement of the degradation potential of laccases [101, 102]. This last decontamination percentage is lower than the percentages reported by other authors [91, 103, 104], although the reaction conditions were different, as Bossa et al. [102] worked with non-purified laccases, with different incubation times, and with other enzymatic activities. Complementary studies demonstrated that laccases synthesized by other *T. gallica* strain was effective in degrading fumonisin B_1 (another frequent mycotoxin in maize and sub-products), achieving a reduction of 60%. This result could lead to the development of a combined strategy for the degradation of more than one toxin.

The conditions during the bioethanol production process, such as fluctuating pH, temperature, and alcohol content, can negatively affect the effectiveness of laccases for AFB_1 degradation. Thus, a study of enzymatic stability was carried out for ensuring effective mycotoxin degradation in samples collected at the fermentation stage. In this way, the enzyme extract containing laccases from *T. gallica* B7-IMICO-RC was evaluated in maize steep liquor with different alcohol concentrations (0.51, 2.45, 8.8, and 14.34°GL) and pH (4.92, 4.39, 4.38, and 4.39, respectively). The results showed that the enzyme is stable at those conditions, supporting its potential application in the previously described industrial process [101].

Subsequently, the experiment was conducted with maize steep liquor, and a 27% reduction in AFB_1 levels was achieved at an enzymatic activity of 5 U/ml and in the presence of 1 mM of vanillic acid. These results are consistent with those reported by Loi et al. [105], who investigated the removal of AFB_1 from ground maize kernels using a purified laccase, achieving a 25% reduction in the concentration of this mycotoxin by employing acetosyringone and dehydroascorbic acid as redox mediators. In our research, although the degradation products of AFB_1 in buffer due to the effect of laccases have not been identified, a cytotoxicity assay was performed on human colorectal adenocarcinoma cells (Caco-2 cell line), and no cytotoxic effects were observed.

This strategy based on the use of fungal laccases could reduce the risk of mycotoxin accumulation in maize sub-products obtained during the bioethanol production process, as well as they could be a useful tool for mitigation of AFs and other mycotoxins in other food and feed products.

6. Conclusions and perspectives

The climate change scenario that the world will face in the coming decades will promote AF production in several food matrices that are vulnerable to infection by toxigenic *A. flavus*. These new climatic conditions challenge us today to urgently develop eco-friendly, cost-effective, and accessible tools for everyone, with the aim of reducing AF contamination levels in raw materials, food and feed intended for human and animal consumption.

In this context, it is necessary to unite efforts of researchers, policymakers, stakeholders, and society as a whole.

In the present chapter, only two approaches are included as cases of study. However, they are just examples of all the work developed by many other researchers around the world, who consider not only efficiency in AF mitigation but also aspects such as environmental impact, optimization of bio-input production, the importance of the degradation product's safety, the reduction of costs and economic losses at different stages of the production processes, and so on. In this sense, advances in science and technology are essential to better understand the problem and its health risks, to prevent those risks, and to apply methods able to eliminate the toxin once it has been synthesized.

Biological control agents to prevent the accumulation of AFs and the complementary strategy of using fungal laccases able to decontaminate AFs without altering food products are promising tools. These technologies have the potential to be integrated into pest management strategies, which include good agricultural practices, predictive models, and physical and chemical methods, among many others.

Additionally, it is crucial that governments implement actions and state policies that ensure food safety worldwide and the commercialization of safe raw materials and food products. The application of necessary training programs should be considered to improve the knowledge, awareness, attitude, and practices of individuals regarding AF mitigation.

Finally, farmers, industry stakeholders, and other participants in the production chains need to be willing to invest in the implementation of various AF mitigation strategies, understanding that these tools will not only bring economic gains but also improve the quality of the food and feed products they produce.

These joint actions will not only guarantee the availability of safe food and feed but also provide the necessary tools to counteract the effects of climate change on the increasing AF contamination levels. All these actions will contribute to food safety, providing the entire population the safe food it demands.

Acknowledgements

The authors thank several agricultural companies from Córdoba province and other regions from Argentina, as well as private producers for kindly providing the commercial fields where the trials were conducted. We also thank the bioethanol producing companies that support our project and provided samples for the assays. We are grateful to several researchers from different local and foreign public and private institutions that contributed with their technical assistance through all these years. These studies were supported by several grants from MYCORED, the Secretary of Science and Technology from the National University of Río Cuarto, the National Research and Technological Council from Argentina (CONICET), and the Research Institute on Mycology and Mycotoxicology (IMICO).

DOI: http://dx.doi.org/10.5772/intechopen.1009018

Author details

María Silvina Alaniz-Zanon, Marianela Bossa, María Laura Chiotta
and Sofía Noemí Chulze*
Research Institute on Mycology and Mycotoxicology (IMICO), National Research and Technological Council from Argentina (CONICET), National University of Río Cuarto (UNRC), Río Cuarto, Córdoba, Argentina

*Address all correspondence to: schulze@exa.unrc.edu.ar

References

[1] Pickova D, Ostry V, Toman J, Malir F. Aflatoxins: History, significant milestones, recent data on their toxicity and ways to mitigation. Toxins. 2021;**13**(6):339. DOI: 10.3390/toxins13060399

[2] Kinyoro IS, Kaale L. Technologies to decontaminate aflatoxins in foods: A review. International Journal of Food Science and Technology. 2024;**59**(10):6783-6796. DOI: 10.1111/ijfs.17435

[3] Magan N, Medina A. Climate change and resilience of biological control agents. In: De Cal A, Melgarejo P, Magan N, editors. How Research Can Stimulate the Development of Commercial Biological Control against Plant Diseases. Progress in Biological Control. Cham: Springer; 2020. pp. 83-93. DOI:10.1007/978-3-030-53238-3_6

[4] Food and Agriculture Organization of the United Nations (FAO). Crop Prospects and Food Situation – Triannual Global Report. Rome, Italy; 2024. Available from: https://openknowledge.fao.org/server/api/core/bitstreams/9256a602-dcee-4af5-8740-302f6f903f7f/content [Accessed: December 24, 2024]

[5] Food and Agriculture Organization of the United Nations (FAO). Crop Prospects and Food Situation – Quarterly Global Report. Rome, Italy; 2022. Available from: https://openknowledge.fao.org/server/api/core/bitstreams/459a8ccc-a90f-45b0-ad8b-24d29ce1abc8/content [Accessed: December 24, 2024]

[6] Eskola M, Kos G, Elliott CT, Hajšlová J, Mayar S, Krska R. Worldwide contamination of food-crops with mycotoxins: Validity of the widely cited 'FAO estimate' of 25%. Critical Reviews in Food Science and Nutrition. 2020;**60**(16):2773-2789. DOI: 10.1080/10408398.2019.1658570

[7] Chulze SN, Alaniz Zanon MS, Taniwaki MH, Tsitsigiannis D, Olsen M, Ortega Beltran A, et al. Aflatoxins in the nut chains: Strategies to reduce their impact on consumer's health and economic losses. World Mycotoxin Journal. 2024;**17**(1):33-56. DOI: 10.1163/18750796-bja10003

[8] Martínez Miranda MM, Vargas del Río LM, Gómez Quintero VM. Aflatoxins: Incidence, impact on health, control and prevention. Bios. 2013;**12**(2):89-109

[9] Hassan HF, Kordahi R, Dimassi H, El Khoury A, Daou R, Alwan N, et al. Aflatoxin B_1 in rice: Effects of storage duration, grain type and size, production site, and season. Journal of Food Protection. 2022;**85**(6):938-944. DOI: 10.4315/JFP-21-434

[10] Elzupir AO, Alamer AS, Dutton MF. The occurrence of aflatoxin in rice worldwide: A review. Toxin Reviews. 2015;**34**(1):37-42. DOI: 10.3109/15569543.2014.984229

[11] Al-Zoreky NS, Saleh FA. Limited survey on aflatoxin contamination in rice. Saudi Journal of Biological Sciences. 2019;**26**(2):225-231. DOI: 10.1016/j.sjbs.2017.05.010

[12] Bhat RV, Krishnamachari KAVR. Follow-up study of aflatoxic hepatitis in parts of western India. Indian Journal of Medical Research. 1977;**66**(1):55-58

[13] Reddy BN, Raghavender CR. Outbreaks of aflatoxicoses in India.

African Journal of Food, Agriculture, Nutrition and Development. 2007;7(5): 1-15. DOI: 10.18697/ajfand.16.2750

[14] Lewis L, Onsongo M, Njapau H, Schurz-Rogers H, Luber G, Kieszak S, et al. Aflatoxin contamination of commercial maize products during an outbreak of acute aflatoxicosis in eastern and Central Kenya. Environmental Health Perspectives. 2005;**113**(12):1763-1767. DOI: 10.1289/ehp.7998

[15] Kamala A, Shirima C, Jani B, Bakari M, Sillo H, Rusibamayila N, et al. Outbreak of an acute aflatoxicosis in Tanzania during 2016. World Mycotoxin Journal. 2018;**11**(3):311-320. DOI: 10.3920/WMJ2018.2344

[16] Popovic R, Radovanov B, Dunn JW. Food scare crisis: The effect on Serbian dairy market. International Food and Agribusiness Management Review. 2017;**20**(1):113-127. DOI: 10.22434/IFAMR2015.0051

[17] Focker M, Van der Fels-Klerx HJ, Oude Lansink AGJM. Financial losses for Dutch stakeholders during the 2013 aflatoxin incident in maize in Europe. Mycotoxin Research. 2021;**37**:139-204. DOI: 10.1007/s12550-021-00429-9

[18] Barros G, Torres A, Palacio G, Chulze S. *Aspergillus* species from section *Flavi* isolated from soil at planting and harvest time in peanut-growing regions of Argentina. Journal of the Science of Food and Agriculture. 2003;**83**(13):1303-1307. DOI: 10.1002/jsfa.1539

[19] Magomya AM, Mbatsav TO. Analysis and health risk evaluation of aflatoxin B_1 levels in groundnut (*Arachis hypogea*) and maize (*Zea mays*) samples from Wukari, Nigeria. European Journal of Theoretical and Applied Sciences. 2023;**1**(4):886-893. DOI: 10.59324/ejtas.2023.1(4).83

[20] Arrus K, Blank G, Abramson D, Clear R, Holley RA. Aflatoxin production by *Aspergillus flavus* in Brazil nuts. Journal of Stored Products Research. 2005;**41**(5):513-527. DOI: 10.1016/j.jspr.2004.07.005

[21] Rapid Alert System for Food and Feed (RASFF). Annual report, 2020-2021-2022. 2022. Available from: https://food.ec.europa.eu/food-safety/rasff_en [Accessed: December 24, 2024]

[22] Tania A, Akram A, Hanif NQ, Ajmal M, Seerat W, Nijabat A, et al. Proximate composition, fungal isolation and contamination of aflatoxin B_1 in chickpea seeds from the Punjab, Pakistan. Natural Product Research. 2023;**37**(19):3314-3322. DOI: 10.1080/14786419.2022.2065674

[23] Ahmadi M, Jahed Khaniki G, Shariatifar N, Molaee-Aghaee E. Investigation of aflatoxins level in some packaged and bulk legumes collected from Tehran market of Iran. International Journal of Environmental Analytical Chemistry. 2022;**102**(16):4804-4813. DOI: 10.1080/03067319.2020.1789614

[24] Alaniz Zanon MS, Bossa M, Chiotta ML, Oddino C, Giovanini D, Cardoso ML, et al. Pre-harvest strategy for reducing aflatoxin accumulation during storage of maize in Argentina. International Journal of Food Microbiology. 2022;**380**:109887. DOI: 10.1016/j.ijfoodmicro.2022.109887

[25] Perrone G, Ferrara M, Medina A, Pascale M, Magan N. Toxigenic fungi and mycotoxins in a climate change scenario: Ecology, genomics, distribution, prediction and prevention of the risk. Microorganisms. 2020;**8**(10):1496. DOI: 10.3390/microorganisms8101496

[26] Shabeer S, Asad S, Jamal A, Ali A. Aflatoxin contamination, its impact and

management strategies: An updated review. Toxins. 2022;**145**(5):307. DOI: 10.3390/toxins14050307

[27] Donnelly R, Elliott C, Zhang G, Baker B, Meneely J. Understanding current methods for sampling of aflatoxins in corn and to generate a best practice framework. Toxins. 2022;**14**(12):819. DOI: 10.3390/toxins14120819

[28] Balan B, Dhaulaniya AS, Kumar M, Kumar M, Kumar P. Aflatoxins in food: Prevalence, health effects, and emerging trends in its mitigation – An updated review. Food Safety and Health. 2024;**2**(1):39-71. DOI: 10.1002/fsh3.12030

[29] Joutsjoki VV, Korhonen HJ. Management strategies for aflatoxin risk mitigation in maize, dairy feeds and milk value chains - Case study Kenya. Food Quality and Safety. 2021;**5**:fyab005. DOI: 10.1093/fqsafe/fyab005

[30] Xu F, Baker RC, Whitaker TB, Luo H, Zhao Y, Stevenson A, et al. Review of good agricultural practices for smallholder maize farmers to minimise aflatoxin contamination. World Mycotoxin Journal. 2021;**15**(2):171-186. DOI: 10.3920/WMJ2021.2685

[31] Alameri MM, Kong ASY, Aljaafari MN, Al AH, Eid K, Al SM, et al. Aflatoxin contamination: An overview on health issues, detection and management strategies. Toxins. 2023;**15**(4):246. DOI: 10.3390/toxins15040246

[32] Brown RL, Menkir A, Chen ZY, Bhatnagar D, Yu J, Yao H, et al. Breeding aflatoxin-resistant maize lines using recent advances in technologies – A review. Food Additives and Contaminants: Part A. 2013;**30**(8):1382-1391. DOI: 10.1080/19440049.2013.812808

[33] Kankam F, Tengey TK, Ndela DN. Evaluation of groundnut genotypes for resistance to early leaf spot disease and Preharvest Aflatoxin contamination. Agricultural and Food Science Journal of Ghana. 2024;**16**(1):1641-1655. DOI: 10.4314/afsjg.v16i1.1

[34] Phan LTK, Tran TM, De Boevre M, Jacxsens L, Eeckhout M, De Saeger S. Impact of season, region, and traditional agricultural practices on aflatoxins and fumonisins contamination in the rice chain in the Mekong Delta. Vietnam. Toxins. 2021;**13**(9):667. DOI: 10.3390/toxins13090667

[35] Chalwe HM, Ngulube M, Njoroge SM, Mweetwa AM, Lungu OI, Phiri EB, et al. The role of manual sorting of raw peanuts to minimize exposure to aflatoxin-contaminated peanuts. Journal of Postharvest Technology. 2019;**7**(3):80-86

[36] Mshanga JP, Makule EE, Ngure FM. Effectiveness of complementary sorting methods in reducing aflatoxin contamination in groundnuts. World Mycotoxin Journal. 2023;**1**(aop):1-15. DOI: 10.1163/18750796-20222830

[37] Mshanga JP, Makule EE, Ngure FM. Physical methods for reduction of aflatoxins exposure in groundnuts in some low-income countries review. Current Research in Nutrition and Food Science. 2023;**11**(2):504-518. DOI: 10.12944/CRNFSJ.11.2.04

[38] Peng Z, Zhang Y, Ai Z, Pandiselvam R, Guo J, Kothakota A, et al. Current physical techniques for the degradation of aflatoxins in food and feed: Safety evaluation methods, degradation mechanisms and products. Comprehensive Reviews in Food Science and Food Safety. 2023;**22**(5):4030-4052. DOI: 10.1111/1541-4337.13197

[39] Sipos P, Peles F, Brassó DL, Béri B, Pusztahelyi T, Pócsi I, et al. Physical and chemical methods for reduction in aflatoxin content of feed and food. Toxins. 2021;**13**(3):204. DOI: 10.3390/toxins13030204

[40] Lagogianni CS, TsitsigiannisDI. Effective chemical management for prevention of aflatoxins in maize. Phytopathologia Mediterranea. 2018;**57**(1):186-198

[41] Montalbano S, Degola F, Bartoli J, Bisceglie F, Buschini A, Carcelli M, et al. The aflatox® project: Approaching the development of new generation, natural-based compounds for the containment of the mycotoxigenic phytopathogen *Aspergillus flavus* and aflatoxin contamination. International Journal of Molecular Sciences. 2021;**22**(9):4520. DOI: 10.3390/ijms22094520

[42] Zhang C, Pan L, Ma J, Yu Q, Yu X, Hussain S, et al. Microencapsulation enhances the antifungal activity of cinnamaldehyde during the period of peanut storage. LWT. 2023;**180**:114657. DOI: 10.1016/j.lwt.2023.114657

[43] Battilani P, Toscano P, Van Der Fels-Klerx HJ, Moretti A, Camardo Leggieri M, Brera C, et al. Aflatoxin B_1 contamination in maize in Europe increases due to climate change. Scientific Reports. 2016;**6**(1):24328. DOI: 10.1038/srep24328

[44] Kaminiaris MD, Leggieri MC, Tsitsigiannis DI, Battilani P. AFLA-PISTACHIO: Development of a mechanistic model to predict the aflatoxin contamination of pistachio nuts. Toxins. 2020;**12**(7):445. DOI: 10.3390/toxins12070445

[45] Li J, Deng J, Bai X, da Graca Nseledge Monteiro D, Jiang H. Quantitative analysis of aflatoxin B_1 of peanut by optimized support vector machine models based on near-infrared spectral features. Spectrochimica Acta Part A: Molecular and Biomolecular Spectroscopy. 2023;**303**:123208. DOI: 10.1016/j.saa.2023.123208

[46] Krska R, Leslie JF, Haughey S, Dean M, Bless Y, McNerney O, et al. Effective approaches for early identification and proactive mitigation of aflatoxins in peanuts: An EU - China perspective. Food Science and Food Safety. 2022;**21**(4):3227-3243. DOI: 10.1111/1541-4337.12973

[47] Voloshchuk N, Irakoze Z, Kang S, Kellogg JJ, Wee J. Three ecological models to evaluate the effectiveness of *Trichoderma* spp. for suppressing aflatoxigenic *Aspergillus flavus* and *Aspergillus parasiticus*. Toxins. 2024;**16**(7):314. DOI: 10.3390/toxins16070314

[48] Moore GG. Practical considerations will ensure the continued success of pre-harvest biocontrol using non-aflatoxigenic *Aspergillus flavus* strains. Critical Reviews in Food Science and Nutrition. 2022;**62**(15):4208-4225. DOI: 10.1080/10408398.2021.1873731

[49] Daigle DJ, Cotty PJ. Formulating atoxigenic *Aspergillus flavus* for field release. Biocontrol Science and Technology. 1995;**5**(2):175-184. DOI: 10.1080/09583159550039891

[50] Bock CH, Cotty PJ. Wheat seed colonized with atoxigenic *Aspergillus flavus*: Characterization and production of a biopesticide for aflatoxin control. Biocontrol Science and Technology. 1999;**9**(4):529-543. DOI: 10.1080/09583159929497

[51] Abbas HK, Accinelli C, Thomas SW. Biological control of aflatoxin contamination in U.S. crops and the

use of bioplastic formulations of *Aspergillus flavus* biocontrol strains to optimize application strategies. Journal of Agricultural and Food Chemistry. 2017;**65**(33):7081-7087. DOI: 10.1021/acs.jafc.7b01452

[52] Dorner JW, Cole RJ, Connick WJ, Daigle DJ, McGuire MR, Shasha BS. Evaluationofbiologicalcontrolformulations to reduce aflatoxin contamination in peanuts. Biological Control. 2003;**26**(3):318-324. DOI: 10.1016/S1049-9644(02)00139-1

[53] Alaniz Zanon MS, Chiotta ML, Giaj-Merlera G, Barros G, Chulze S. Evaluation of potential biocontrol agent for aflatoxin in Argentinean peanuts. International Journal of Food Microbiology. 2013;**162**(3):220-225. DOI: 10.1016/j.ijfoodmicro.2013.01.017

[54] Accinelli C, Abbas HK, Vicari A, Shier WT. Aflatoxin contamination of corn under different agro-environmental conditions and biocontrol applications. Crop Protection. 2014;**63**:9-14. DOI: 10.1016/j.cropro.2014.04.021

[55] Weaver MA, Abbas HK, Jin X, Elliott B. Efficacy of water-dispersible formulations of biological control strains of *Aspergillus flavus* for aflatoxin management in corn. Food Additives and Contaminants: Part A. 2016;**33**(2):346-351. DOI: 10.1080/19440049.2015.1129071

[56] Accinelli C, Abbas HK, Vicari A, Shier WT. Evaluation of recycled bioplastic pellets and a sprayable formulation for application of an *Aspergillus flavus* biocontrol strain. Crop Protection. 2015;**72**:9-15. DOI: 10.1016/j.cropro.2015.02.020

[57] Dorner JW, Horn BW. Separate and combined applications of nontoxigenic *Aspergillus flavus* and *A. Parasiticus* for biocontrol of aflatoxin in peanuts. Mycopathologia. 2007;**163**:215-223. DOI: 10.1007/s11046-007-9004-0

[58] Alaniz Zanon MS, Barros GG, Chulze SN. Non-aflatoxigenic *Aspergillus flavus* as potential biocontrol agents to reduce aflatoxin contamination in peanuts harvested in northern Argentina. International Journal of Food Microbiology. 2016;**321**:63-68. DOI: 10.1016/j.ijfoodmicro.2016.05.016

[59] Mauro A, Garcia-Cela E, Pietri A, Cotty PJ, Battilani P. Biological control products for aflatoxin prevention in Italy: Commercial field evaluation of atoxigenic *Aspergillus flavus* active ingredients. Toxins. 2018;**10**(1):30. DOI: 10.3390/toxins10010030

[60] Doster MA, Cotty PJ, Michailides TJ. Evaluation of the atoxigenic *Aspergillus flavus* strain AF36 in pistachio orchards. Plant Disease. 2014;**98**(7):948-956. DOI: 10.1094/PDIS-10-13-1053-RE

[61] Ain NU. Advancing sustainable agriculture: Bioinputs and solid-state fermentation innovations for eco-friendly farming. International Journal of Agriculture and Sustainable Development. 2024;**6**(2):90-101

[62] DeClerck FAJ, Koziell I, Benton T, Garibaldi LA, Kremen C, Maron M, et al. A whole earth approach to nature-positive food: Biodiversity and agriculture. In: Von Braun J, Afsana K, Fresco LO, Hassan MHA , editors. Science and Innovations for Food Systems Transformation. Cham: Springer; 2023. pp. 469-496. DOI: 10.1007/978-3-031-15703-5_25

[63] Trabelsi D, Mhamdi R. Microbial inoculants and their impact on soil microbial communities: A review. BioMed Research International.

2013;**2013**(1):863240. DOI: 10.1155/2013/863240

[64] Lewis MH, Carbone I, Luis JM, Payne GA, Bowen KL, Hagan AK, et al. Biocontrol strains differentially shift the genetic structure of indigenous soil populations of *Aspergillus flavus*. Frontiers in Microbiology. 2019;**10**:1738. DOI: 10.3389/fmicb.2019.01738

[65] de Miranda SL, de Moura JB, Lopes Filho LC, Teixeira MF, de Castro PJ. Bioinputs: A sustainable alternative to traditional pesticide cultivation. Observatório De La Economía Latinoamericana. 2023;**21**(12):24777-24816. DOI: 10.55905/oelv21n12-073

[66] Reyes-Calderón A, Pérez-Uribe S, Ramos-Delgado AG, Ramalingam S, Oza G, Parra-Saldívar R, et al. Analytical and regulatory considerations to mitigate highly hazardous toxins from environmental matrices. Journal of Hazardous Materials. 2022;**423**:127031. DOI: 10.1016/j.jhazmat.2021.127031

[67] Ministerio de Agricultura Pesca y Alimentación (MAGyP). 2024. Available from: https://www.magyp.gob.ar/sitio/areas/estimaciones/_archivos/estimaciones/240000_2024/240100_Enero/240118_Informe%20mensual%20al%2018_01_2024.pdf [Accessed: December 24, 2024]

[68] Garrido CE, Hernández Pezzani C, Pacin A. Mycotoxins occurrence in Argentina's maize (*Zea mays* L.), from 1999 to 2010. Food Control. 2012;**25**(2):660-665. DOI: 10.1016/j.foodcont.2011.11.043

[69] Barros GG, Torres AM, Rodriguez MI, Chulze SN. Genetic diversity within *Aspergillus flavus* strains isolated from peanut-cropped soils in Argentina. Soil Biology and Biochemistry. 2006;**38**(1):145-152. DOI: 10.1016/j.soilbio.2005.04.028

[70] Barros G, Torres A, Chulze S. *Aspergillus flavus* population isolated from soil of Argentina's peanut-growing region. Sclerotia production and toxigenic profile. Journal of the Science of Food and Agriculture. 2005;**85**(14):2349-2353. DOI: 10.1002/jsfa.2257

[71] Chiotta ML, Oviedo S, Barros G, Torres A, Chulze SN. Potential biocontrol agent for aflatoxins in peanuts in Argentina. In: XII International IUPAC Symposium on Mycotoxins and Phycotoxins; 21-25 May 2007. Istanbul, Turkey: IUPAC (International Union of Pure and Applied Chemistry); 2007

[72] Alaniz Zanon MS. Reducción de la entrada de aflatoxinas en la cadena agroalimentaria maní. Biocontrol basado en la exclusión competitiva [Doctoral Thesis]. Río Cuarto, Córdoba, Argentina: Universidad Nacional de Río Cuarto; 2016

[73] Alaniz Zanon MS, Clemente MP, Chulze SN. Characterization and competitive ability of non-aflatoxigenic *Aspergillus flavus* isolated from the maize agro-ecosystem in Argentina as potential aflatoxin biocontrol agents. International Journal of Food Microbiology. 2018;**277**:58-63. DOI: 10.1016/j.ijfoodmicro.2018.04.020

[74] Rhein P. Control biológico de aflatoxinas en maíz: Impacto sobre la diversidad fúngica en suelo y efectividad frente a un escenario de cambio climático [Graduate Thesis]. Río Cuarto, Córdoba, Argentina: Universidad Nacional de Río Cuarto; 2024

[75] Nada S, Nikola T, Bozidar U, Ilija D, Andreja R. Prevention and practical strategies to control mycotoxins in the wheat and maize chain. Food Control. 2022;**136**:108855. DOI: 10.1016/j.foodcont.2022.108855

[76] Loi M, Fanelli F, Liuzzi VC, Logrieco AF, Mulè G. Mycotoxin

biotransformation by native and commercial enzymes: Present and future perspectives. Toxins. 2017;**9**(4):111. DOI: 10.3390/toxins9040111

[77] Eisa NA, Ali FM, El-Habbaa GM, Abdel-Reheem SK, Abou-El-Ela MF. Pulsed electric field technology for checking aflatoxin production in cultures and corn grains. Egyptian. Journal of Phytopathology. 2020;**31**:75-86

[78] Vanga SK, Wang J, Orsat V, Raghavan V. Effect of pulsed ultrasound, a green food processing technique, on the secondary structure and *in vitro* digestibility of almond milk protein. Food Research International. 2020;**137**:109523. DOI: 10.1016/j.foodres.2020.109523

[79] Hojnik N, Modic M, Walsh JL, Žigon D, Javornik U, Plavec J, et al. Unravelling the pathways of air plasma induced aflatoxin B_1 degradation and detoxification. Journal of Hazardous Materials. 2021;**403**:123593. DOI: 10.1016/j.jhazmat.2020.123593

[80] Ismail A, Gonçalves BL, de Neeff DV, Ponzilacqua B, Coppa CFSC, Hintzsche H, et al. Aflatoxin in foodstuffs: Occurrence and recent advances in decontamination. Food Research International. 2018;**113**:74-85. DOI: 10.1016/j.foodres.2018.06.067

[81] Kumar V, Bahuguna A, Ramalingam S, Dhakal G, Shim JJ, Kim M. Recent technological advances in mechanism, toxicity, and food perspectives of enzyme-mediated aflatoxin degradation. Critical Reviews in Food Science and Nutrition. 2022;**62**(20):5395-5412. DOI: 10.1080/10408398.2021.2010647

[82] Sun X, Sun C, Zhang X, Zhang H, Ji J, Liu Y, et al. Aflatoxin B_1 decontamination by UV-mutated live and immobilized *Aspergillus Niger*. Food Control. 2016;**61**:235-242. DOI: 10.1016/j.foodcont.2015.09.017

[83] Liu M, Zhang X, Luan H, Zhang Y, Xu W, Feng W, et al. Bioenzymatic detoxification of mycotoxins. Frontiers in Microbiology. 2024;**15**:1434987. DOI: 10.3389/fmicb.2024.1434987

[84] Liu DL, Yao DS, Liang R, Ma L, Cheng WQ, Gu LQ. Detoxification of aflatoxin B_1 by enzymes isolated from *Armillariella tabescens*. Food and Chemical Toxicology. 1998;**36**(7):563-574. DOI: 10.1016/S0278-6915(98)00017-9

[85] Li CH, Li WY, Hsu IN, Liao YY, Yang CY, Taylor MC, et al. Recombinant aflatoxin-degrading F420H2-dependent reductase from *mycobacterium smegmatis* protects mammalian cells from aflatoxin toxicity. Toxins. 2019;**11**(5):259. DOI: 10.3390/toxins11050259

[86] Afsharmanesh H, Perez-Garcia A, Zeriouh H, Ahmadzadeh M, Romero D. Aflatoxin degradation by *Bacillus subtilis* UTB1 is based on production of an oxidoreductase involved in bacilysin biosynthesis. Food Control. 2018;**94**:48-55. DOI: 10.1016/j.foodcont.2018.03.002

[87] Zhou M, Fakayode OA, Ren M, Li H, Liang J, Yagoub AEGA, et al. Laccase-catalyzed lignin depolymerization in deep eutectic solvents: Challenges and prospects. Bioresources and Bioprocessing. 2023;**10**(1):21. DOI: 10.1186/s40643-023-00640-9

[88] Wang X, Qin X, Hao Z, Luo H, Yao B, Su X. Degradation of four major mycotoxins by eight manganese peroxidases in presence of a dicarboxylic acid. Toxins. 2019;**11**(10):566. DOI: 10.3390/toxins11100566

[89] Loi M, Renaud JB, Rosini E, Pollegioni L, Vignali E, Haidukowski M, et al. Enzymatic transformation of aflatoxin B_1 by Rh_DypB peroxidase and characterization of the reaction products. Chemosphere. 2020;**250**:126296. DOI: 10.1016/j.chemosphere.2020.126296

[90] Shao H, Su X, Wang Y, Zhang J, Tu T, Wang X, et al. Oxidative degradation and detoxification of multiple mycotoxins using a dye-decolorizing peroxidase from the white-rot fungus *Bjerkandera adusta*. LWT. 2024;**206**:116597. DOI: 10.1016/j.lwt.2024.116597

[91] Alberts JF, Gelderblom WCA, Botha A, Van Zyl WH. Degradation of aflatoxin B_1 by fungal laccase enzymes. International Journal of Food Microbiology. 2009;**135**(1):47-52. DOI: 10.1016/j.ijfoodmicro.2009.07.022

[92] Loi M, Fanelli F, Zucca P, Liuzzi VC, Quintieri L, Cimmarusti MT, et al. Aflatoxin B_1 and M_1 degradation by Lac2 from *Pleurotus pulmonarius* and redox mediators. Toxins. 2016;**8**(9):245. DOI: 10.3390/toxins8090245

[93] Mani P, Kumar VTF, Keshavarz T, Sainathan Chandra T, Kyazze G. The role of natural laccase redox mediators in simultaneous dye decolorization and power production in microbial fuel cells. Energies. 2018;**11**(12):3455. DOI: 10.3390/en11123455

[94] Loi M, Fanelli F, Cimmarusti MT, Mirabelli V, Haidukowski M, Logrieco AF, et al. *In vitro* single and combined mycotoxins degradation by Ery4 laccase from *Pleurotus eryngii* and redox mediators. Food Control. 2018;**90**:401-406. DOI: 10.1016/j.foodcont.2018.02.032

[95] Abudabos AM, Al-Atiyat RM, Khan RU. A survey of mycotoxin contamination and chemical composition of distiller's dried grains with solubles (DDGS) imported from the USA into Saudi Arabia. Environmental Science and Pollution Research. 2017;**24**:15401-15405. DOI: 10.1007/s11356-017-9130-2

[96] Hernández O, Lopez A, Nazareno MA, García EM, Reineri P, Fissolo H, et al. Effect of supplementation with corn DDGS on intake and ruminal fermentation parameters by beef steers fed a tropical grass hay. Journal of Animal Science. 2018;**96**:437-438

[97] Mohammadi Shad Z, Venkitasamy C, Wen Z. Corn distillers dried grains with solubles: Production, properties, and potential uses. Cereal Chemistry. 2021;**98**(5):999-1019. DOI: 10.1002/cche.10445

[98] Zhang Y, Caupert J. Survey of mycotoxins in U.S. distiller's dried grains with solubles from 2009 to 2011. Journal of Agricultural and Food Chemistry. 2012;**60**(2):539-543. DOI: 10.1021/jf203429f

[99] Oplatowska-Stachowiak M, Haughey SA, Chevallier OP, Galvin-King P, Campbell K, Magowan E, et al. Determination of the mycotoxin content in distiller's dried grain with solubles using a multianalyte UHPLC-MS/MS method. Journal of Agricultural and Food Chemistry. 2015;**63**(43):9441-9451. DOI: 10.1021/acs.jafc.5b03844

[100] Mallmann CA, Simões CT, Kobs Vidal J, Rosa Da Silva C, De Lima Schlösser LM, Araújo De Almeida CA. Occurrence and concentration of mycotoxins in maize dried distillers' grains produced in Brazil. World Mycotoxin Journal. 2021;**14**(3):259-268. DOI: 10.3920/WMJ2020.2669

[101] Bossa M, Monesterolo NE, M Del P M, Rhein P, Chulze SN,

Alaniz-Zanon MS, et al. Fungal laccases and fumonisin decontamination in co-products of bioethanol from maize. Toxins. 2024;**16**(8):350. DOI: 10.3390/toxins16080350

[102] Bossa M, Alaniz-Zanon MS, Monesterolo NE, M Del P M, Coria YM, Chulze SN, et al. Aflatoxin decontamination in maize steep liquor obtained from bioethanol production using laccases from species within the Basidiomycota phylum. Toxins. 2024;**16**(1):27. DOI: 10.3390/toxins16010027

[103] Zeinvand-Lorestani H, Sabzevari O, Setayesh N, Amini M, Nili-Ahmadabadi A, Faramarzi MA. Comparative study of *in vitro* prooxidative properties and genotoxicity induced by aflatoxin B_1 and its laccase-mediated detoxification products. Chemosphere. 2015;**135**:1-6. DOI: 10.1016/j.chemosphere.2015.03.036

[104] Scarpari M, Bello C, Pietricola C, Zaccaria M, Bertocchi L, Angelucci A, et al. Aflatoxin control in maize by *Trametes versicolor*. Toxins. 2014;**6**(12):3426-3437. DOI: 10.3390/toxins6123426

[105] Loi M, De Leonardis S, Ciasca B, Paciolla C, Mulè G, Haidukowski M. Aflatoxin B_1 degradation by Ery4 laccase: From *in vitro* to contaminated corn. Toxins. 2023;**15**(5):310. DOI: 10.3390/toxins15050310

Chapter 4

Different Detection, Quantification, and Inhibition Techniques for Aflatoxin Content in Food, Crop, and Feed

Nethra Puttaswamy

Abstract

Aspergillus flavus is a soil-borne fungi, found commonly in tropical and subtropical climates. The most common crops infected by *Aspergillus flavus* during the growing period are maize, groundnut, chili, cottonseed, etc. Improper management of the crops during the growing period leads to the contamination of the fungi. These fungi release aflatoxins, which are furanocoumarin-derived compounds and among the most potent mycotoxins contaminating field crops. Various studies were conducted for the detection and decontamination of aflatoxin from the food, crop, or feed, and also various management strategies were adopted to overcome aflatoxin contamination by eliminating fungus. But all these strategies were restricted only for detecting and reducing aflatoxin contamination. Modern approaches including genomic and metabolomic studies have been utilized to explore the molecular mechanisms of resistance to aflatoxin contamination. Recently, the rapid development of emerging nanotechnology scaled up its dimension of thinking toward the application of various types of nanomaterials for the detection and elimination of aflatoxin contents. One important application is the development of nanosensors, which further helped to improve its sensitivity. Many nanomaterials have been extensively applied in antifungal, aflatoxin adsorption, inhibition, and detoxification process. Hence, nanotechnology in the future could be an important tool for eliminating aflatoxin contamination in various commodities.

Keywords: aflatoxin, *Aspergillus flavus*, molecular genetics, nanotechnology, aflatoxin detection, elimination

1. Introduction

Aflatoxin is a secondary metabolite and an important derivative of mycotoxin produced by various fungi. It is one of the most significant and harmful toxins, affecting various crops, food products, and feed. As a consequence, it has a profound detrimental effect on animal and human health [1, 2]. The studies have reported that aflatoxin is a potent mutagenic and carcinogenic compound, which upon exposure

Aflatoxin	Fungal species	Host/affected entity
AFLB1 and AFLB2	*Aspergillus flavus, Aspergillus parasiticus, A. arachidicola, A. nomius, A. oryzae, A. tamarii, A. ochraceoroseus, A. bombycis, A. pseudotamarii, A. parvisclerotigenus, etc.*	Maize, peanuts, pea, rice, sorghum, sunflower seeds, spices, cottonseed, figs, dairy products, oilseed rape, maize flour, meat, peanut butter, fruit juices (guava apple)
AFLG1 and G2	*A. nomius, A. arachidicola, A. bombycis, A. parasiticus, A. pseudotamarii A. versicolor, A. terreus, A. toxicarius, A. minisclerotigenes*	Maize, maize flour, meat, cottonseed, dairy products, fruit juices (guava, apple) Oilseed rape, peanuts, peanut butter, pea, figs, pistachio, rice, sorghum, sunflower seed, spices
AFLM1, AFLM2	These are the hydroxylated metabolites of AFL B1 and AFLB2,	Meat, milk, and dairy products
GM1	These are the hydroxylated metabolites of AFL G1 is produced naturally by *Aspergillus parasiticus* and *Aspergillus flavus.*	Milk and dairy products

Table 1.
Aflatoxin affecting fungal species and the affected commodities.

causes serious health hazards affecting the brain, heart, liver, and kidneys in humans [3]. Aflatoxin contamination drastically reduces the export quality of many commercially grown crops across the globe. According to FAO (Food and Agriculture Organization), it has been reported that more than 25% contamination of the food is majorly by mycotoxins [4]. *Aspergillus flavus* and *Aspergillus parasiticus* are the two common fungi that produce aflatoxins. Other fungal species such as *A.nomius, A pseudotomarii*, *A. parvisclerotigenus*, and *A bombycis*, etc., also produce aflatoxin [5]. Currently, more than eighteen types of aflatoxins (AFL) have been identified from various fungal sources and the most common and important ones are AFLB1, AFLB2, AFLG1, and AFLG2 as listed in **Table 1**. These suffices were given depending on their characteristic absorbance and emittance of light at different wavelengths. AFLB1 and AFLB2 show characteristic blue fluorescence at 425 nm, while AFLG1 and AFLG2 show characteristic green fluorescence at 540 nm [4, 6, 7]. *Aspergillus spp*. such as *A. nomius, A. parasiticus, Aspergillus bombycis, etc.,* produce all four types of aflatoxins, viz. AFLB1, AFLB2, AFLG1, and AFLG2; whereas, *Aspergillus flavus, Aspergillus rambellii,* and *Aspergillus ochraceoroseus* produce AFLB1 and AFLB2. The other *Aspergillus* species such as *A. pseudotamarii, and Emericell astellata* produce only AFLB1 [8]. The AFM1 and AFLM2 types, which are the derivative of AFLB1 and AFLB2 respectively have been found in the animal milk and urine (**Table 1**) [9].

2. Life cycle of *Aspergillus spp. and its* mode of infection

Aspergillus flavus is a soil-borne fungus that is seen more in tropical and subtropical climates where latitudes are between 16° and 35°. They mostly survive as conidia or sclerotia in the soil for more than a year and form mycelia in the plant tissues when infected. These conidia or sclerotia remain in the soil during unfavorable environmental situations and upon the onset of the favorable conditions, they form mycelia and then into conidiophores which get dispersed into the atmosphere and infect a wide range of plants. The mode of replication of *Aspergillus flavus* is largely by asexual reproduction. Few studies have also reported that sexual reproduction is also possible among the compatible groups of the strain [10]. It has high genetic diversity as compared to other *Aspergillus species*. Biotic and abiotic stresses, as well as post-harvest practices such as improper management during storage conditions of the crops, lay the foundation for its infection, colonization, and toxin production [11]. The crops that are infected with *A. flavus* are maize, groundnut, chili, cottonseed, etc., during their growing period, while the crops that are most susceptible at post-harvest stages are rice, wheat, and sorghum [12]. These fungi produce high levels of toxins in the infected seeds at the time of harvest with high protein and lipid content [13]. The toxin-producing strains are categorized into S and L types. S strains produce high levels of aflatoxins with numerous sclerotia (diameter of <400 μm), whereas L strains produce large sclerotia with a diameter of >400 μm [14]. The other *Aspergillus* species such as *A. sojae* and *A. oryzae* which are known as domesticated counterparts of *A. parasiticus* and *A flavus* respectively, do not produce aflatoxins, although they possess the homologs of the aflatoxin biosynthesis pathway genes [15]. This may be due to its genetic recombination caused during sexual reproduction which is naturally occurring in nature [16].

3. Management of aflatoxin contamination

New advanced technologies were adopted in the recent years to mitigate and control aflatoxin contamination in food, grain, and feed. Several recent research activities oriented toward reducing aflatoxin content through several approaches have been discussed in this book chapter with separate headings.

3.1 Physical method of aflatoxin decontamination

Physical separation of the aflatoxin-contaminated product (kernels, seeds, and nuts) from the non-contaminated product is the first method of aflatoxin reduction. Cleaning, sorting, and hand-picking are the most reliable techniques which are safe to use. Studies have reported that hand sorting of maize kernels could detect 6% AFB1 as compared to other methods [17]. All these manually operated methods take a long time and have low success rates in preventing aflatoxin contamination. Heat inactivation or thermal treatments, irradiation, density segregation, etc., are the other common methods to control aflatoxin contamination. Studies have shown that roasting almonds at 200°C significantly reduces aflatoxin levels. The shelf life of the food items can be increased by treating it with UV radiation which degrades the fungal cell wall and thereby suppresses its growth [18]. Different thermal and ionization treatments can inhibit aflatoxin content from 10 to 100% depending upon the type of commodity used. 100–150°C heat treatment for 90 min showed a significant reduction in AFB1 content in soybean [19]. Vegetables and fruits when autoclaved at 120°C for 30 min, can reduce the aflatoxin content from 9–39%, whereas, peanuts when autoclaved for 80–90 min can completely inhibit aflatoxin levels [20]. However, subjecting the food crops to high thermal, ionization, and UV treatments, its nutritional quality would be adversely affected.

Owing to the adverse effects on the nutritional properties, the other alternative approach is by nonthermal technologies such as high pressure of 500 MPa for 5–8 min could successfully decrease the aflatoxin contents in water samples by 61–87% [21]. Cold plasma treatment reduces aflatoxin by up to 90–95% in different nuts and grains [22]. It is found to be a more cost-effective and eco-friendly treatment since it does not affect the quality of the feed or the grains [23]. Gamma irradiation could reduce aflatoxin contamination in fruits and vegetables by up to 60% [24]. It not only reduces the fungal population but also reduces the mycotoxin content in the infected grains. Gamma irradiation dosage ranging from 1 to 10 kGy causes nearly a 69.8% reduction in fungal growth and a 94.5% reduction in the mycotoxin content in corn kernels [25, 26]. But frequent exposure to gamma radiation may cause slight changes in the chemical composition of the food which can alter the nutrient content of some food. A cost-effective multispectral analyzer was used to detect the aflatoxin content in corn kernels. The hyperspectral imaging and infrared spectroscopy were also been in practice to detect fungal infection and aflatoxin content [27]. Pulsed electric field is a short pulse of electric current given at the range of 80 kV/cm to 100 V/cm, which alters the fungal cell permeability. The study showed that a pulsed electric field can reduce both aflatoxin B2 and G1 contents in grape juices as well as in water [28]. Pulsed light technology was found to be an efficient method of decontamination of bacteria, fungi, viruses, etc., from the food and other materials [29]. The adsorbents, which include synthetic polymers, diatomaceous earth, zeolites, bentonite, zeolite, sodium calcium aluminosilicates, activated charcoal, etc., were used in poultry feeds, which at the time of intake, the toxins get attached to these adsorbents and thereby preventing them from mixing into the bloodstream and thereby removes from their body [18, 24, 30]. These adsorbents were also demonstrated in vegetable oils also [31, 32]. Although, these compounds are used as an adsorbent product which can reduce the bioavailability of mycotoxins, but, in practice, the toxins cannot be completely adsorbed by these products. The drawback of using adsorbents is that it may cause unspecific binding of the nutrients (**Table 2**).

Physical method		
Method	**Commodity [References]**	**% reduction efficiency**
Washing	Corn [33, 34]	90–97
Dehulling and polishing	Corn [33, 34], Rice [35]	92, 88–92
Thermal treatment	Soybean [19], Peanut [36], Wheat [37]	50–90, 42–81, 57–80
Near infrared radiation, UV light treatment	Peanuts [38], Rice [39], Milk [28]	65–100, <99, 14–17
Gamma radiation	Soybean [40], Wheat, Rice [41]	22–69, 27–65, 62–76
Pulse Light treatment	Rice kernel [42]	39–90
Cold/nonthermal plasma treatment	Corn [43], Peanuts [44]	62–82, 23–38
Chemical method		
Ammonification	Milk [45]	79–90
Ozone treatment	Wheat [46], corn [47, 48], poultry feed [49]	85–95, 79–95, 86
Organic and inorganic acids	Black pepper, mixed feed, grains [49]	< 92

Table 2.
Physical and chemical methods for aflatoxin removal from food, crop, and feed.

3.2 Chemical method of aflatoxin decontamination

This method involves various inorganic and organic acids such as citric acid, tartaric acid, lactic acid, propionic acid, etc., which has shown good results for the control of aflatoxin. Citric acid treatment has shown nearly 86–92% reduction in AFB1 content in the feed, while lactic acid has shown a moderate reduction of 67%. The chemical treatment with sodium bisulfite shows nearly 28–68% inhibition in aflatoxin content depending on the differential techniques used [50, 51]. The oxidizing agent like ammonium persulfate showed nearly 31–51% reduction in AFB1 contents [52, 53]. Sodium hydrosulfite was also found to be effective in reducing aflatoxin content (96–100%) in black pepper when applied at a range from 0.25 to 2% [54]. Various studies highlighted the use of ozone in reducing the aflatoxin content up to 66–95% in cereal grains, pulses, soybeans, peanuts, etc. [24] Ozone molecules target directly mycotoxin inhibition without affecting the quality of food [55, 56]. Studies have reported that ozone when used at a concentration of 50 mg/L with a flow rate of 5 L/min for 60 h, destroyed AFB1 content in peanuts by 89.4% [57]. Similarly, the aflatoxins in peanuts were readily destroyed at moisture content of 5% (w/w), when treated with ozone at the concentration of 6 mg/L for 30 min at room temperature. Treatment with alkaline compounds, salts, and acids showed reduction in aflatoxin content up to 18–51% [58]. Recent studies highlighted the application of hexane and chloroform in inhibiting the aflatoxin production. Antioxidants like butylated hydroxytoluene, and butylated hydroxyanisole also showed tremendous inhibition of *A. flavus* which ultimately reduced the aflatoxin content [18]. The major drawback of the chemical method of decontamination is that it may impair the taste and appearance of food. The residue remaining in the food after chemical treatment may be harmful to humans.

3.3 Biological method of aflatoxin decontamination

Various microbes release secondary metabolites into the soil ecosystem, making it crucial to understand their ecological impact due to higher heterogeneity of the soil environment [59]. One useful tool to prevent aflatoxin contamination in the soil is by using different bacterial and fungal isolates present in the natural ecosystem which are antagonists to the strains producing aflatoxin. The most prominent method is to use the strains of *Aspergillus flavus* which are naturally atoxigenic. Morphologically, the atoxigenic are L -type strains that produces more sclerotia but with very less or completely devoid of aflatoxin. This may be due to genetic variations caused by the deletion of the genes that are involved in the aflatoxin biosynthesis pathway [60]. These strains were successfully used as a biocontrol agent for many years to control the growth of toxigenic strains of *Aspergillus* in the field [61, 62]. These biocontrol agents require strong validation to assess its stability, adaptation, and efficacy under different environmental conditions. There are various techniques used for its characterization such as marker-based PCR analysis which helps to analyze the genes undergoing deletion to differentiate between toxigenic and atoxigenic strains [63]. The first commercial biocontrol agent, AF36 strain was registered and used successfully in the USA to control aflatoxin contamination in cotton seeds. Atoxigenic strains used in the fields of peanut, cotton, and corn showed nearly 70–90% reduction in aflatoxin production [64]. The atoxigenic strain NRRL21882 of *Aspergillus flavus* and NRRL21369 of *A. parasiticus*, when applied to the peanut field, showed effective control on aflatoxin production both during pre-harvest and post-harvest stages. It was commercially used as a biopesticide in the name of Afla-guard [65]. Similarly, BN

30 atoxigenic strain in Africa, showed successful control of aflatoxin production in maize fields [18]. There was a 95% reduction in aflatoxin content in peanuts by using atoxigenic strains as reported in Australia [66]. The atoxigenic strain of *Aspergillus flavus* namely AF051 in China was found to control aflatoxin production effectively up to 99% in peanut fields [18]. In the southern US, the four-year study data on maize showed the successful inhibition of *A. flavus* up to 65–94% by using atoxigenic strains K49 and CT3. Similarly, the two-year study conducted in Northern Argentina demonstrated the efficient use of atoxigenic strains AR27, AR100G, and AFCHG2 in the groundnut field [67].

The application of biopesticides is streaming in different parts of the globe where the countries have come forward for its registration. But the lacuna in the study conducted was restricted to evaluate only the pathogens as biocontrol agents were limited only to a few years of study trials, and were not formulated as a bioproduct [60]. But some studies also showed that most of the biofungicides do not reduce aflatoxin content, but indeed inhibit the mycelial or conidial growth of *A. flavus* [68].

Apart from fungus, there are various bacterial and yeast strains that also show aflatoxin inhibition. Studies have shown that several yeast strains such as *Saccharomyces cerevisiae* (RC008 and RC016), *Candida maltose*, *Pichia anomala*, etc., showed a drastic inhibition of *Aspergillus* spp. and a reduction in the aflatoxin content. But still, they need to be validated under open field conditions [60]. *Trichoderma* spp., such as *Trichoderma auroviride* and *Trichoderma longibrachiatum* also showed a reduction in aflatoxin content by up to 80%. *Penicillium* spp., *P. chrysogenum,* and *P. nalgiovense* are used as a biocontrol agent against various phytopathogenic fungi [60]. Many different bacterial strains such as *Lactobacilii, Pseudomonas, Ralstonia, Streptomyces, Bacillus*, etc., also showed tremendous aflatoxin inhibition [69]. The main advantage of this method is that it shows high specificity and can completely detoxify the samples under suitable conditions, making the product safe and harmless. But it also has certain drawbacks such as mass production of the microbes for commercial application is a huge challenge since it is very difficult to control the microbial performance which can even turn out to be unsafe on the new products.

Various studies have reported that co-cultivation has become one of the powerful tools to reduce or prevent the aflatoxin contamination in food, feed, and grains [70]. *Rhizopus oligosporus*, prevented or destroyed the synthesis of AFB1 toxin produced from *Aspergillus* flavus [71]. *Bacillus subtilis* ANSB060 isolated from fish gut successfully detoxified aflatoxin. Studies reported that by adding *Bacillus subtilis* ANSB060 to the aflatoxin-contaminated feed of the laying hens, broilers and dairy cows could inhibit the aflatoxin contamination [72–74].

A latest study has reported the use of Lactic acid bacteria (LAB) for degradation of aflatoxins in food and feed. LAB have shown to possess antifungal activity and hence turned out to be a potential for bio preservation. Among different strains of LAB, *Lactobacillus plantarum* is notably the best-known strain for fungal inhibitory activity. LAB degrades aflatoxin by producing various antifungal metabolites such as organic acids, phenolic compounds, cyclic dipeptides, decanoic acid derivatives, hydrogen peroxide, etc. [75, 76]. Hence *Lactobacillus* strains have been shown to have potential application in food industries including dairy products, animal feed, and others. However, further studies are needed to understand deeply the effect of LAB strains on the nutritional quality of food, feed, and the ability to combat multiple combinations of toxins before they are commercially applied in Industrial mass production.

4. Techniques for detecting aflatoxin-producing strains

The various detection methods were used for aflatoxin contamination which include cultural and molecular-based techniques. The details are given below in the text as well its merits and demerits in **Table 3**.

4.1 Culture-based technique

Different culture media were used to identify aflatoxin-producing fungal strains. These media include Yeast Extract sucrose medium, Aflatoxin producing Ability media, Coconut Milk Agar media, Coconut Agar Medium, etc. When the fungal strain was grown on the suitable media and observed under the wavelength of 365 nm, the formation of fluorescent ring surrounding the colonies illustrates the presence of an aflatoxin-producing strain and can able to differentiate from the atoxigenic strains. The major drawback of this technique is that it only differentiates toxigenic and atoxigenic strains but cannot quantify the actual aflatoxin content [77].

4.2 Immunochemical method

This method includes ELISA (Enzyme-linked immunosorbent assay) and Radioimmunoassay (RIA) which use antigens and antibodies depending upon their specificities. ELISA is among the most rapid and reliable methods for detecting aflatoxin, particularly in food products. In many research and medical laboratories, ELISA kits are commercially available for aflatoxin detection and quantification at very minute concentrations [78]. The radioimmunoassay is based on the radiolabeled antigen which reacts with the specific antibody. This method is highly efficient but sensitive because of the use of radiolabeled antigen which is dangerous and hence has limited use [79].

4.3 Biosensor-based technique

Different biosensors are used which include optical immunosensors, electrochemical immunosensor, microfluidic sensor method, sensor array method, etc., to detect aflatoxin contamination in crops and various food products. It is based on the principle of antigen and antibody interaction which is detected through a signal transducer [80–82]. The optical immunosensors rely largely on the detection of antibody-antigen interface. They are used to detect proteins, peptides, biomarkers, nucleic acids, etc. Surface plasmon resonance (SPR) device and optical waveguide light-mode spectroscopy (OWLS) are among the few important sensors. The electrochemical immunosensors consist of an amplifier that recognizes the signals produced by the integration of antibodies and which can be quantified. They are more reliable for detection of AFM1 in milk at a concentration ranging from 0.01 to 1 μg/L [82]. The microfluidic sensor method is a paper-based microfluidic device, where the samples are allowed to run on this device, and a quick color change will be observed. This method is suitable for the detection of AFM1 and AFB1 [81]. It is a semiconducting device that uses electrochemical signals that is converted into data and can be evaluated. It was successfully used to detect AFM1 in milk samples [82].

4.4 Chromatographic methods

It is based on the physical interaction between mobile and stationary phase. There are different chromatographic techniques used such as thin layer chromatography

Techniques	Advantages	Limitations
Culture-based techniques	Different culture media are used which differentiate between toxigenic and atoxigenic strains.	This procedure cannot quantify aflatoxin concentration.
Marker-based technique	Different markers and real-time PCR assays are used to amplify genes that are involved in aflatoxin biosynthesis pathways.	This technique only validates the genes involved in aflatoxin biosynthesis, but cannot detect or prevent aflatoxin contamination.
Immunochemical method		
ELISA	Works on the principle of antigen -antibody interaction which is a rapid, reliable, and relatively cheaper method for aflatoxin detection.	Depends on the binding specificities of antigen and antibody.
Radioimmunoassay	The principle is the same as ELISA. This technique is highly sensitive, which quantifies even at very low concentration of the sample.	Not commonly used because of the radioactive labeled antigens.
Biosensor-based techniques		
Optical immunosensors	It allows the real-time detection of toxins in the sample.	The device is huge and heavy. Application under field condition is not possible.
Electrochemical immunosensor	It is cost-effective, simple, and time-saving.	Application under field condition is not possible.
Microfluidic sensor method	This method is quick, precise, and cost-effective.	
Sensor array method	It is a rapid method for detecting toxins in the sample.	
Chromatographic methods		
Thin layer chromatography (TLC)	Easy to operate, simple, and cost-effective.	Not very precise. Harmful reagents are used, and highly sensitive. Expert technicians are required as the procedure is cumbersome.
High-performance liquid chromatography (HPLC)	Has good repeatability and low detection time.	Very expensive and needs precise operation by an expert.
Ultra performance liquid chromatography (UPLC)	More advanced than HPLC and highly sensitive readings can be obtained.	Very expensive and needs precise operation by an expert.
Liquid chromatography and mass spectrometry (LC-MS)	More advanced and highly précised readings can be obtained.	Expensive instrument and complex operation procedures.

Table 3.
Different detection techniques for identifying aflatoxin contamination.

(TLC), high-performance liquid chromatography (HPLC), and liquid chromatography-mass spectrometry (LC-MS) for the detection and quantification of aflatoxins in various food crops such as maize, peanuts, figs, coffee beans, spices, etc., including milk and dairy products [83]. In TLC, the mobile phase consists of a mixture of acetonitrile, methanol, and water while the stationary phase consists of cellulose, silica, or alumina, which is immobilized on a glass or plastic matrix. The mobile phase moves on the stationary phase along with the sample. TLCs were used to detect various types of mycotoxins. However, the measurement is not accurate and precise and hence other advanced methods like HPLC and LC-MS were preferred for aflatoxin detection. The studies have reported that these techniques are highly sensitive and accurate and hence preferred for the quantification of aflatoxins in various food and food grains [83]. But these methods are labor-intensive and require skilled operation.

4.5 Spectroscopic methods

The spectroscopic methods include fluorescence spectrophotometry which uses different fluorescence by emitting energy at specific wavelengths, and Frontier infrared spectroscopy which uses infrared radiation to detect and quantify aflatoxin concentration [84].

4.6 Molecular techniques for aflatoxin detection

The aflatoxin resistance mechanisms acquired by the host during host-pathogen interaction are divided into three types namely Invitro seed colonization (IVSC), pre-harvest aflatoxin contamination (PAC), and aflatoxin production (AP) [85]. To understand the aflatoxin resistance, various modern biotechnological tools are used to identify the promising lines that are resistant to all these mechanisms [86]. The transcriptomic, proteomic, and metabolomic studies were used to identify different biochemical pathways and the genes that are involved in aflatoxin biosynthesis. Besides this, it also helps in identifying different proteins which are synthesized during fungal infection. Next-generation sequencing technologies have accelerated the large genomic studies in a very affordable manner [87]. QTL analysis (quantitative trait loci) helps in identifying the linked markers for aflatoxin resistance. The complete genome sequencing of hosts and pathogens helps in identifying the novel genes. The use of sophisticated tools such as RNA-sequencer provides insight into the molecular mechanism of toxin production by the pathogens and resistance mechanism acquired by different crops [88–93]. All these studies have helped the breeders and researchers to dwell into the development of transgenic free maize [94] and groundnut [95]. Different gene silencing mechanisms such as post-transcriptional gene silencing and RNA interference help in reducing the aflatoxin content in groundnut by complete silencing of aflatoxin-producing genes such as *aflP, aflR, aflS, aflC*, etc. Overexpression of antifungal plant defensins (*Msdef1*) using recombinant DNA technology also helps in reducing aflatoxin production [95]. But the major drawback of this technique is that they do not provide any heritable resistance in the genotype.

5. Nanotechnological intervention in aflatoxin control

To reduce the aflatoxin contamination in various crops, food products, and in animal feed, the application of nanotechnology plays a very important role. The use of different nanomaterials has been explored at four different levels as mentioned below.

5.1 Mold inhibition

The studies from the past research confirm that the materials at the nanoscale level exhibit an antimicrobial property which has been widely explored in medical research. The antibacterial nanoparticles are used in antibiotics against various pathogenic bacteria. However, the antifungal properties have not been much explored because of the differences in the structural and functional properties between bacteria and fungi. The latest findings revealed the use of antifungal nanoparticles in combating aflatoxin by inhibiting *Aspergillus spp.* This method uses metal nanoparticles which are stable and can have positive effects through green synthesis routes using plant, animal sources, and micro-organisms which show less toxicity and are environmentally friendly [96]. ZnO nanoparticles have been reported to inhibit *Botrytis cinerea* and *Penicillium expansum*. ZnO NP treatment showed deformation of the fungal hyphae which was observed through a scanning electron microscope. The possible reason suggested that ZnO nanoparticle (NP) produces reactive oxygen species (ROS) which led to the damage of the lipid bilayer of the cell membrane and thereby breakdown of the cell [97]. The application of AgNP at 45 ppm reduction in aflatoxin production by up to 80% in *Aspergillus niger* and *Pencillium chrysogenum* [98]. These studies infer that the nanoparticle having antimicrobial properties needs to be explored further in aflatoxin elimination.

5.1.1 Aflatoxin adsorption

The activated charcoal was earlier used as an adsorbent for mycotoxin elimination. Nowadays the most promising successor of this is the engineered carbon nanomaterials which are being used for mycotoxin elimination because of its large surface area per weight, high adsorptive properties, excellent stability, inertness, and colloidal stability. Fullerene, nanofiber, nanodiamonds, graphene, graphene oxide, and nanotubes have great potential as novel adsorbents of mycotoxins because of its crystalline structure and C-C covalent bonds which makes them strong, elastic, and good conductors of electricity [99]. Fullerene is one such prominent nanomaterial whose adsorption behavior is much higher than that of activated carbon. Preliminary investigation showed that there was a significant decrease in the aflatoxin concentration in the media when its was treated with fullerenol nanoparticles, it also showed reduced mycelial biomass in the media [100]. Nanodiamonds exhibit a high adsorptive capacity for AFB1 through electrostatic interactions [101]. The numerous oxygen functional groups present on the magnetic graphene oxide nanoparticle enabled the interaction with mycotoxins [102]. Chitosan nanoparticles has shown promising results with 70% efficacy in mycotoxin adsorption and elimination since it is nontoxic, having low immunogenicity, and is biodegradable [103]. Studies have shown that glutaraldehyde crosslinked chitosan nanoparticles also showed promising adsorption ability for aflatoxin B1 [104].

5.1.2 Aflatoxin elimination

Many recent studies have shown that the green synthesized nanoparticles such as cerium, oxides of zinc, iron, titanium, silver, gold, selenium, etc., have shown a unique antioxidant property since they are enriched with natural compounds to increase their donor activity [105–107]. Many metal oxide and metal hydroxide nanoparticles have shown inhibitory effects on various pathogens, particularly on bacteria and fungi. Many studies have shown that ZnO NPs possess an outstanding antifungal activity without any photoactivation. Navale [108], reported that ZnO NPs showed antimicrobial activity against two pathogenic bacteria i.e., *Staphylococcus aureus* and *Salmonella typhimurium* and also against two plant pathogenic fungi i.e.,

Aspergillus fumigatus and *A. flavus* [108]. CuNPs also showed superior antifungal activity against *Fusarium oxysprorum, Curvularia lunata, and Alternaria alternata* [109]. The biosynthesized AgNPs also showed outstanding inhibition of mycotoxigenic fungal strains including *Alternaria alternata, A.ochraceus, Aspergillus flavus,* and *Fusarium solani* [110]. In addition to this, various studies were carried out on other NPs such as MgO NPs, FeO NPs, and TiO_2 NPs for its antifungal and antibacterial activities. A very recent study conducted by Mukherjee [111], who prepared N, F Co-doped TiO_2 NPs with the nano-size limit of 200–300 nm as an antifungal agent, which could efficiently interact with the fungal cell wall/membrane causing damage to it through the generation of ROS. Although many studies have conducted on different nanoparticles with antimicrobial properties, however, their effectiveness against mycotoxin elimination has not been completely explored. More studies should come up in this direction.

5.1.3 Aflatoxin detoxification

Detoxification of mycotoxins, particularly aflatoxin, is a huge challenge in all the agriculture sectors. As previously discussed in chapters 3.1, 3.2, and 3.3, there are many strategies for aflatoxin detoxification such as physical, chemical, and biological methods. However, these methods still have some limitations with regard to the residual problem, and use of toxic chemicals for aflatoxin adsorption which may cause environmental pollution and may require a long period of growth [112]. Owing to all these limitations, many recent studies suggested the use of oxidation technology through photocatalytic degradation which was found to exhibit unique properties in the detoxification of aflatoxins. This method fetches low cost, is environmentally friendly, easy to handle with no pollution [113]. There are plenty of nanomaterials such as Fe_2O_3, ZnO composites with graphene, TiO_2, etc., which has become an attractive hotspot for aflatoxin detoxification due to its photocatalytic properties [112, 114]. A novel nanosized g-C_3N_4 sheets were prepared with the size range from 50 to 150 nm and which showed enhanced photocatalytic degradation of AFB1 under visible light

Fungal species	Plant/ microbial extract	Nanoparticle with average size	Inhibition dose	Reference
Aspergillus niger and *A. flavus*	*Cissus quadrangularis*	CuO (30 nm)	1000 ppm	[115]
Aspergillus fumigatus and *Candida albicans*	*Bacillus* spp.	Selenium (140 nm)	100 µg/mL	[116]
Fusarium	*Chaetomium globosum*	Silver (15 nm)	500 mg/L	[117]
Rhizopus sp and *Aspergillus sp.*	leaf extract of *Aloe vera*	Silver (70 nm)	100 µL /M	[118]
Aspergillus flavus	*Penicillium citrinum*	Silver (54 nm)	4000 ppm	[119]
Fusarium, Aspergillus and *Candida*	*Arthroderma fulvum*	Silver (15 nm)	1 mg/mL	[120]
Aspergillus ochraceus	*Penicillium expansum* and *Aspergillus terreus*	Silver (20 nm)	3 and 9 g/100 mL	[121]

Table 4.
Green synthesized nanoparticle as an antifungal agent.

as compared to the bulk g-C_3N_4. This was attributed to its larger surface with good charge separation efficiency (**Table 4**) [122].

5.2 Nanomaterials used for HPLC assays

The aflatoxin contamination in the food can be detected using various analysis systems such as HPLC and LC-MS/MS, where various types of nanoparticles are used for detection. The metal and metal oxide nanoparticles such as Fe_3O_4 MNPs were used for the extraction of aflatoxin B1, B2, G1, and G2 in cereals and nut samples which was coupled with HPLC and fluorescence-based assays [123]. Although the HPLC-based assays for the detection and quantification of aflatoxin were found to be highly sensitive and accurate, still the method is very laborious, time-consuming, and requires skilled operators [124]. Hence a fast and reliable method for aflatoxin detection is urgently required.

5.3 Nanomaterials-based immunoassays

Immunoassay depends on antigen-antibody interaction and the detection can be assessed with simple analysis devices. This is one of the most popular methods for rapid and efficient analysis in the laboratory. However, with the advent of nanotechnology and due to numerous unique properties of nanomaterials, immunoassays have achieved progress in the detection of aflatoxins [125]. The nanomaterials such as AuNPs, AgNPs, MNPs, etc., provide good biocompatibility with biomolecule immobilization, leading to high signal amplification. Quantum dots which are semiconductors having broad absorption and narrow emission spectrum with unique photoluminescence properties can be employed as a signal label for the immunoassays of aflatoxin [124]. Li and his co-workers developed a fluorometric lateral flow immunoassay, where he used Au/Ag NPs which help in signal amplification to detect mycotoxins like AFB1, ZEN, and DON in cereal crops [126]. In recent years, different nanomaterials-based immunoassays have been used with high-quality antibodies to detect aflatoxins, but it still suffers from intrinsic limits such as complex preparation, time consumption, and high cost which can be replaced with a promising alternative to antibodies with molecular-based aptamers and biosensors for effective detection.

5.4 Nanomaterials-based aptasensors

Aptamers are a group of peptide and nucleic acid molecules with a distinct recognition element that undergoes a special reaction with various analytes. This unique property of aptamers made them to be used in the development of aptasensors [127]. Scientists have integrated many different nanomaterials such as metal and metal oxide NPs, magnetic NPs, COFs, MOFs, and carbon-based nanoparticles such as CNTs, graphene, etc., into the aptasensors to increase its selectivity and sensitivity [126, 128]. Nanomaterial-based aptasensor play an important role in signal generation [129], signal amplification [130], fluorescence quencher [131], etc., in aflatoxin detection. In recent years, the advanced nanoenzyme-based aptasensor for aflatoxin detection has emerged [132]. For example, AuNPs with peroxidase-mimicking activity was used for the detection of ZEN mycotoxin [133]. Similarly, Huang and his co-workers developed a new colorimetric aptasensor based on $MnCO_2O_4$ nanozyme activity for OTA analysis in corn samples [134]. Zhu also developed a new colorimetric aptasensor to detect aflatoxin B1 and OTA in agricultural products [135].

5.5 Nano biosensors for aflatoxin detection

5.5.1 Metal nanomaterials as biosensors

Metal nanomaterials have a strong adsorption characteristic, which does not affect the normal biological activities and hence were used to detect various enzyme activities. Besides this, metal nanomaterials have unique optical and electrical properties which are used in food analysis. They are also highly compatible with various biomolecules such as antibodies, enzymes, aptamers, etc.; hence are highly recommended for detecting food contaminants. The phenomenal property of the emission and absorption spectrum of metal nanomaterials due to its quantum size effect, makes them more effective in qualitative and quantitative analysis of aflatoxins [136–138]. Researchers have used various types of nanomaterials for the detection of aflatoxin in different commodities. For example, Zhang prepared a semiquantitative immunochromatographic strip that can be used for aflatoxin detection visually [139]. Song developed the LFIA method for quantitative and semiquantitative determination of different types of mycotoxins such as aflatoxin B1, ZEA (zearalenone), DON (Vomitoxin), etc., in foodgrains [140]. Anfossi and co-workers prepared a strip for quantitative analysis of aflatoxins [141]. Arati et al., developed an electrochemical immunoassay method for AFB1 detection using gold nanoparticles [142].

All these studies infer that the nano biosensors provide a rapid screening of aflatoxin in various food and agricultural commodities because of its high sensitivity, near accuracy with a simple operating procedure.

5.5.2 Metal oxide nanomaterials as biosensors

Metal oxide and hydroxide nanoparticles have higher stability than metal nanoparticles used in aflatoxin detection. This is due to their high mechanical strength, large surface area, and high electronic and catalytic properties, which has regarded them as a prominent substance for detecting various target samples [118, 143]. Singh and his workers developed an electrochemical sensor by immobilizing Sm_2O_3 nanorods and nickel nanoparticles on the electrode surface which can detect up to 10–700 pg./ml aflatoxin B1 in the food sample [144]. Chauhan developed an immunosensor which is made of reusable electrochemical quartz crystal microbalance (QCM) for the detection of AFB1 [145].

5.5.3 Carbon nanomaterials as biosensors

The carbon-based nanomaterials such as carbon nanotubes, fullerenes, carbon nanofibers, carbon quantum dots, graphene, and their derivatives have laid the strong foundation for the analysis and detection of aflatoxins in various crop and food commodities because of its unique physicochemical properties. Gan and his workers constructed an electrochemiluminescence (ECL) device using magnetic graphene oxide and antibody-labeled quantum dot, carbon nanotube (CNT) composite for detection of AFM1 in milk [146]. This implies that CNTs have good adsorption characteristics that help in faster amplification of ECL signals for effective detection of aflatoxin. Zhang used SWCNTs/chitosan nanocomposite to design an electrochemical immunoassay for AFB1 detection

Type of nanomaterials	NPs	Receptor molecules	Target	Sample	Detection signal	Reference
Metal nanomaterials	AuNPs	Antibody/PEDOT	AFB1	Corn	Electrochemical signal	[148]
	Ni NPs	Antibody	AFB1	Corn	Electrochemical signal	[149]
	GNRs	Antibody	AFB1	Peanut	Colorimetric signal	[145]
Metal oxides and hydroxides	Fe_3O_4 nanoparticles	Antibody	AFB1	Food	Electrochemical signal	[150]
Carbon nanomaterials	CNTs	Antibody/CdTe QDs	AFM1	Milk	Electrochemiluminescence signal	[147]
	CNTs	Antibody/ PDDA	AFB1	Rice	Electrochemical signal	[151]
	SWCNTs	Antibody/_-NP	AFB1	Corn meal	Electrochemical signal	[96]
	MWCNTs	Antibody/[BMIM]PF6	AFB1	Olive oil	Electrochemical signal	[152]
	GO	Aptamer	AFM1	Milk	Electrochemiluminescence signal	[153]
	rGO	Aptamer/ polyaniline	AFB1	Wine	Electrochemical signal	[154]
	Graphene	Antibody/ PANI	AFB1	Rice	Electrochemical signal	[155]
	GQDs	Antibody/_-cyclodextrin	AFM1	Milk	Electrochemical signal	[156]
Other nanomaterials	MBs	Antibody	AFB1	Corn, Maize	Colorimetric signal	[157, 158]
	MBs	Aptamer/DNA-scaffolded AgNCs	AFB1	Wheat, rice, corn	Fluorescent signal	[153]
	MNPs	Aptamer/ PAPDI	AFB1	Maize	Fluorescent signal	[154]
	QDs	Aptamer/QDs	AFB1	Rice, peanut	Fluorescent signal	[155]

Note: NPs: nanoparticles; PEDOT: poly(2,3-dihydrothieno-1,4-dioxin); AFM1: aflatoxin M1; GNRs: gold nanorods; CNTs: Carbon nanotubes; PDDA: poly dimethyl diallyl ammonium chloride; PAPDI: perylene probe; QD: Quantum dots.

Table 5.
Different nanomaterials for aflatoxin detection.

[147]. The other carbon nanomaterials such as carbon dots, nano horns, mesoporous carbon, and nanospheres have also been used for aflatoxin detection (**Table 5**).

Although there are various applications with nanomaterials for combating aflatoxin contamination, but still many more nanomaterials need to be explored and further developed.

5.6 Challenges and future research directions for nanotechnology in aflatoxin control

The advent of nanotechnology has made great progress in the use of nanomaterials in aflatoxin control, detection, and elimination, but still faces great challenges in its application as discussed below:

- Although, various detection methods are used for aflatoxin contamination, but still, many improvements need to be framed with respect to the cost of production, low toxicity, and mass production of nanomaterials without adverse effects on the environment. The reproducibility of some of the nanomaterials is very difficult to achieve due to the complexity of its structures. Therefore, the efficient novel nanomaterials which has better porosity, good reproducibility, and control over its shape and surface interactions need to be further explored.

- While using nanomaterials as biosensors, it should possess high specificity in binding to the sample matrix to avoid nonspecific signals in the detection of aflatoxin.

- The development of ultrasensitive nanosensors which can detect various types of mycotoxins occurring in food grains, food and feeds simultaneously are very much required.

- The automatic and portable small equipment which are highly sensitive and reliable in its on-spot detection of aflatoxin need to be developed.

6. Conclusion and prospective

Aflatoxin is one of the group of mycotoxins produced by different species of *Aspergillus*. It gets contaminated in food and feeds unpredictably and unavoidably leading to adverse health effects both in animals and humans which causes huge economic losses to the agriculture and food industries. Management of aflatoxin contamination is a great challenge and has raised an alarming signal worldwide. With the advent of new technologies, it has enabled to tackle the aflatoxin contamination at the early stages itself. Molecular approaches such as omics, genomics, transcriptomics, and metabolomics have helped to understand the structure and the biosynthetic pathways of aflatoxin. There are various pre-harvest and post-harvest management practices such as physical, chemical, and biological methods which are found to be effective in aflatoxin decontamination. There are many sophisticated detection techniques used such as ELISA, immunoassays, HPLC and LC-MS methods, and chromatographic and spectrophotometric methods for aflatoxin detection in food, feed, and crops which have turned out to be effective.

Although there are significant detection techniques available, they have shown some limitations in their accuracy and specificity. Amazingly in the emerging new era, nanotechnology has rapidly scaled up in all the fields of science. The potential use of nanomaterials in aflatoxin detection and inhibition has marked worldwide attention. One important application that has reached the milestone is the development of nanosensors, which increased the sensitivity and specificity of sample detection. Hence most of the research focused on understanding the science and the application of nanomaterials for quantitative detection and inhibition of aflatoxins. For this, a large variety of nanomaterials are being used such as carbon nanomaterials, metal, metal oxide, and metal hydroxide nanomaterials. But, at present most of the nano biosensor devices used for detection of aflatoxin are still at the laboratory research stage and it is difficult to detect samples in real time as quickly and conveniently as possible. Hence further studies need to be done on the analytical devices. Although many nanomaterials have been extensively used as an antimicrobial, aflatoxin adsorption, and detoxification process, but still its application is in the infant stage to address the health outcomes and ensure food safety. Hence expanding the detection methods using various nanomaterials by simplifying the detection equipment is the direction of future research.

Acknowledgements

I acknowledge the University of Agricultural Sciences, Dharwad, Karnataka, India and also IntechOpen for providing the opportunity to write this book chapter.

Conflicts of interest

I Nethra P declare that I do not have any conflict of interest for publication.

Author details

Nethra Puttaswamy
Department of Crop Physiology, College of Agriculture, University of Agricultural Sciences, Dharwad, Karnataka, India

*Address all correspondence to: nethrap@uasd.in

References

[1] Peles F, Sipos P, Gyori Z, Pfliegler WP, Giacometti F, Serraino A, et al. Adverse effects, transformation, and channeling of aflatoxins into food raw materials in livestock. Frontiers in Microbiology. 2019;**10**:2861

[2] Ráduly Z, Szabó L, Madar A, Pócsi I, Csernoch L. Toxicological and medical aspects of aspergillus-derived mycotoxins entering the feed and food chain. Frontiers in Microbiology. 2019;**10**:2908

[3] Kumar P, Mahato DK, Kamle M, Mohanta TK, Kang SG. Aflatoxins: A global concern for food safety, human health and their management. Frontiers in Microbiology. 2017;7:2170

[4] Luo S, Du H, Kebede H, Liu Y, Xing F. Contamination status of major mycotoxins in agricultural product and food stuff in Europe. Food Control. 2021;**127**:108-120

[5] Ahmad MM, Ahmad M, Ali A, Hamid R, Javed S, Abdin MZ. Detection of *Aspergillus flavus* and *Aspergillus parasiticus* from aflatoxin-contaminated peanuts and their differentiation using PCR-RFLP. Annals of Microbiology. 2014;**64**:1597-1605

[6] Benkerroum N. Aflatoxins: Producing-molds, structure, health issues and incidence in southeast Asian and sub-Saharan African countries. International Journal Environmental Research and Public Health. 2020;**17**:1215

[7] Abdin M, Ahmad MM, Javed S. Advances in molecular detection of Aspergillus: An update. Archives of Microbiology. 2010;**192**:409-425

[8] Coppock RW, Christian RG, Jacobsen BJ. Aflatoxins. In: Gupta RC, editor. Veterinary Toxicology. 3rd ed. Cambridge, MA, USA: Academic Press; 2018. pp. 983-994

[9] Lalah JO, Omwoma S, Orony DAO. Aflatoxin B1: Chemistry, environmental and diet sources and potential exposure in human in Kenya. In: Aflatoxin B1 Occurrence, Detection and Toxicological Effects. Norderstedt, Germany: BoD–Books on Demand; 2020

[10] Horn BW, Moore GG, Carbone I. Sexual reproduction in *Aspergillus flavus*. Mycologia. 2009;**101**:423-429

[11] Varshney RK, Pandey MK, Bohra A, Singh VK, Thudi M, Saxena RK. Toward the sequence-based breeding in legumes in the post-genome sequencing era. Theoretical and Applied Genetics. 2019;**132**:797-816

[12] Bertioli DJ, Cannon SB, Froenicke L, Huang G, Farmer AD, Cannon EK, et al. The genome sequences of *Arachis duranensis* and *Arachis ipaensis*, the diploid ancestors of cultivated peanut. Nature Genetics. 2016;**48**:438-446

[13] Molyneux RJ, Mahoney N, Kim JH, Campbell BC. Mycotoxins in edible tree nuts. International Journal of Food Microbiology. 2007;**119**:72-78

[14] Cotty PJ. Virulence and cultural characteristics of two *Aspergillus flavus* strains pathogenic on cotton. Phytopathologia. 1989;**79**:808-814

[15] Payne GA, Nierman WC, Wortman JR, Pritchard BL, Brown D, Dean RA. Whole genome comparison of *Aspergillus flavus* and *Aspergillus oryzae*. Medical Mycology. 2006;**44**:9-11

[16] Horn BW, Gell RM, Singh R, Sorensen RB, Carbone I.

Sexual reproduction in *Aspergillus flavus* sclerotia: Acquisition of novel alleles from soil populations and uniparental mitochondrial inheritance. PLoS One. 2016;**11**(1):0146169

[17] Matumba L, Van Poucke C, Njumbe Ediage E, De Saeger JB, . Effectiveness of hand sorting, flotation/washing, dehulling and combinations thereof on the decontamination of mycotoxin-contaminated white maize. Food Additives and Contaminants. 2015;**6**:960-969

[18] Yin Y, Yan L, Jiang J, Ma ZH. Biological control of aflatoxin contamination of crops. Journal of Zhejiang University Science. 2008;**9**:787-792

[19] Lee J, Her J, Lee G. Reduction of aflatoxins (B1, B2, G1, and G2) in soybean-based model systems. Food Chemistry. 2015;**189**:45-51

[20] Samarajeewa U, Sen A, Cohen M, Wei C. Detoxification of aflatoxins in foods and feeds by physical and chemical methods. Journal of Food Protection. 1990;**53**:489-501

[21] Pallarés N, Berrada H, Tolosa J, Ferrer E. Effect of high hydrostatic pressure (HPP) and pulsed electric field (PEF) technologies on reduction of aflatoxins in fruit juices. Food Science and Technology. 2021;**142**:110-120

[22] Misra NN, Yadav B, Roopesh MS. Cold plasma for effective fungal and mycotoxin control in foods: Mechanisms, inactivation effects, and applications. Comprehensive Reviews in Food Science and Food Safety. 2019;**18**:106-120

[23] Hojnik N, Cvelbar U, Tavcar-Kalcher G, Walsh JL, Križaj I. Mycotoxin decontamination of food: Cold atmospheric pressure plasma versus "classic" decontamination. Toxins. 2017;**9**:151

[24] Sipos P, Peles F, Brassó DL, Béri B, Pusztahelyi T, Pócsi I, et al. Physical and chemical methods for reduction in aflatoxin content of feed and food. Toxins. 2021;**13**:204

[25] Markov K, Mihaljevic B, Domijan M, Pleadin J, Delaš F, Frece J. Inactivation of aflatoxigenic fungi and the reduction of aflatoxin B1 in vitro and in situ using gamma irradiation. Food Control. 2015;**54**:79-85

[26] Serra MS, Pulles MB, Mayanquer FT, Vallejo MC, Rosero MI, Ortega JM, et al. Evaluation of the use of gamma radiation for reduction of aflatoxin B1 in corn (*Zea mays*) used in the production of feed for broiler chickens. Journal of Agricultural Chemistry and Environment. 2018;7:21-33

[27] Eisa NA, Ali FM, El-Habbaa GM, Abdel-Reheem SK, Abou-El-Ella MF. Pulsed electric field technology for checking aflatoxin production in cultures and corn grains. Egyptian Journal of Phytopathology. 2020;**31**:75-86

[28] Hassan FF, Hussein HZ. Detection of aflatoxin M1 in pasteurized canned milk and using of UV radiation for detoxification. International Journal of Advances in Chemical Engineering and Biological Sciences. 2017;**4**:130-133

[29] Elmnasser N, Guillou S, Leroi F, Orange N, Bakhrouf A, Federighi M. Pulsed-light system as a novel food decontamination technology: A review. Canadian Journal of Microbiology. 2007;7:813-821

[30] Tahir NI, Hussain S, Javed M, Rehman H, Shahzady TG, Parveen B, et al. Nature of aflatoxins: Their extraction, analysis, and control. Journal of Food Safety. 2018;**38**:2561

[31] Ji J, Xie W. Detoxification of aflatoxin B1 by magnetic graphene composite adsorbents from contaminated oils. Journal of Hazardous Materials. 2020;**381**:120915

[32] Ji J, Xie W. Removal of aflatoxin B1 from contaminated peanut oils using magnetic attapulgite. Food Chemistry. 2021;**339**:128072

[33] Fandohan P, Zoumenou D, Hounhouigan DJ, Marasas WFO, Wingfield MJ, Hell K. Fate of aflatoxins and fumonisins during the processing of maize into food products in Benin. International Journal of Food Microbiology. 2005;**98**:249-259

[34] Mutungi C, Lamuka P, Arimi S, Gathumbi J, Onyango C. The fate of aflatoxins during processing of maize into muthokoi—A traditional Kenyan food. Food Control. 2008;**19**:714-721

[35] Castells M, Ramos AJ, Sanchis V, Marín S. Distribution of total aflatoxins in milled fractions of hulled rice. Journal of Agricultural and Food Chemistry. 2007;**55**:2760-2764

[36] Arzandeh S, Jinap S. Effect of initial aflatoxin concentration, heating time and roasting temperature on aflatoxin reduction in contaminated peanuts and process optimisation using response surface modelling. International Journal of Food Science and Technology. 2011;**46**:485-491

[37] Hwang H, Lee G. Reduction of aflatoxin B1 contamination in wheat by various cooking treatments. Food Chemistry. 2006;**98**:71-75

[38] Shen MH, Singh R. Effect of rotating peanuts on aflatoxin detoxification by ultraviolet C light and irradiation uniformity evaluated by AgCl-based dosimeter. Food Control. 2021;**120**:107-533

[39] Ferreira CD, Lang GH, da Silva LI, da Silva TN, Hoffmann JF, Ziegler V, et al. Postharvest UV-C irradiation for fungal control and reduction of mycotoxins in brown, black, and red rice during long-term storage. Food Chemistry. 2021;**339**:127810

[40] Zhang ZS, Xie QF, Che LM. Effects of gamma irradiation on aflatoxin B1 levels in soybean and on the properties of soybean and soybean oil. Applied Radiation and Isotopes. 2018;**139**:224-230

[41] Mohamed NF, El-Dine RSS, Kot MAM, Saber A. Assessing the possible effect of gamma irradiation on the reduction of aflatoxin B1, and on the moisture content in some cereal grains. American Journal of Biomedical Science and Research. 2015;**7**:33-39

[42] Wang B, Mahoney NE, Pan Z, Khir R, Wu B, Ma H, et al. Effectiveness of pulsed light treatment for degradation and detoxification of aflatoxin B1 and B2 in rough rice and rice bran. Food Control. 2016;**59**:461-467

[43] Shi H, Ileleji K, Stroshine RL, Keener K, Jensen JL. Reduction of aflatoxin in corn by high voltage atmospheric cold plasma. Food Bioprocess and Technology. 2017;**10**:1042-1052

[44] Iqdiam BM, Abuagela MO, Boz Z, Marshall SM, Goodrich-Schneider R, Sims CA, et al. Effects of atmospheric pressure plasma jet treatment on aflatoxin level, physiochemical quality, and sensory attributes of peanuts. Food Processing and Preservation. 2020;**44**(e14305):72

[45] Phillips TD. Dietary clay in the chemoprevention of aflatoxin-induced disease. Toxicological Sciences. 1999;**52**:118-126

[46] Savi GD, Piacentini KC, Scussel VM. Ozone treatment efficiency in Aspergillus and Penicillium growth inhibition and mycotoxin degradation of stored wheat grains (*Triticum aestivum* L.). Food Processing and Preservation. 2015;**39**:940-948

[47] McKenzie KS, Kubena LF, Denvir AJ, Rogers TD, Hitchens GD, Bailey RH, et al. Aflatoxicosis in Turkey poults is prevented treatment of naturally contaminated corn with ozone generated by electrolysis. Poultry Science. 1998;**77**:1094-1102

[48] Luo X, Wang R, Wang L, Li Y, Bian Y, Chen Z. Effect of ozone treatment on aflatoxin B1 and safety evaluation of ozonized corn. Food Control. 2014;**37**:171-176

[49] Torlak E, Akata I, Erci F, Uncu AT. Use of gaseous ozone to reduce aflatoxin B1 and microorganisms in poultry feed. Stored Product Research. 2016;**68**:44-49

[50] Colovic R, Puvacˇa N, Cheli F, Avantaggiato G, Greco D, Đuragic O, et al. Decontamination of mycotoxin contaminated feedstuffs and compound feed. Toxins. 2019;**11**:617

[51] Altug T, Yousef AE, Marth EH. Degradation of aflatoxin B1 in dried figs by sodium bisulfite with or without heat, ultraviolet energy or hydrogen peroxide. Journal of Food Protection. 1990;**53**:581-582

[52] Rushing B, Selim MI. Aflatoxin B1: A review on metabolism, toxicity, occurrence in food, occupational exposure, and detoxification methods. Food and Chemical Toxicology. 2019;**124**:81-100

[53] Shi H, Stroshine R, Ileleji K. Determination of the relative effectiveness of four food additives in degrading aflatoxin in distillers' wet grains and condensed distillers solubles. Journal of Food Protection. 2017;**80**:90-95

[54] Jalili M, Jinap S. Role of sodium hydrosulphite and pressure on the reduction of aflatoxins and ochratoxin A in black pepper. Food Control. 2012;**27**:11-15

[55] Tiwari BW, Brennan CS, Curran T, Gallagher E, Cullen PJ, Donnell CP. Application of ozone in grain processing. Journal of Cereal Science. 2010;**51**:248-255

[56] Zhu F. Effect of ozone treatment on the quality of grain products. Food Chemistry. 2018;**264**:358-366

[57] Diao E, Hou H, Chen B, Shan C, Dong H. Ozonolysis efficiency and safety evaluation of aflatoxin B1 in peanuts. Food Chemistry and Toxicology. 2013;**55**:519-525

[58] Jalili M, Jinap S, Son R. The effect of chemical treatment on reduction of aflatoxins and ochratoxin A in black and white pepper during washing. International Society for Mycotoxicology. 2011;**28**:485-493

[59] Fouche T, Claassens S, Maboeta M. Aflatoxins in the soil ecosystem: An overview of its occurrence, fate, effects and future perspectives. Mycotoxin Research. 2020;**36**(3):303-309

[60] Ren X, Zhang Q, Zhang W, Mao J, Li P. Control of Aflatoxigenic molds by antagonistic microorganisms: Inhibitory behaviors, bioactive compounds, related mechanisms, and influencing factors. Toxins. 2020;**12**:2

[61] Cotty P, Bayman P. Competitive exclusion of a toxigenic strain of *Aspergillus flavus* by an atoxigenic strain. Phytopathology. 1993;**83**:1283-1287

[62] Okun DO, Khamis FM, Muluvi GM, Ngeranwa JJ, Ombura FO, Yongo MO, et al. Distribution of indigenous strains of atoxigenic and toxigenic *Aspergillus flavus* and *Aspergillus parasiticus* in maize and peanuts agro-ecological zones of Kenya. Agriculture & Food Security. 2015;**4**:1-10

[63] Callicott K, Cotty P. Method for monitoring deletions in the aflatoxin biosynthesis gene cluster of *Aspergillus flavus* with multiplex PCR. Letters in Applied Microbiology. 2015;**60**:60-65

[64] Cotty PJ. Development of *Aspergillus flavus* AF36; 2005

[65] Dorner J, Lamb MC. Development and commercial use of afla-guard®, an aflatoxin biocontrol agent. Mycotoxin Research. 2006;**22**:33-38

[66] Pitt J, Hocking AD. Mycotoxins in Australia: Biocontrol of aflatoxin in peanuts. Mycopathologia. 2006;**162**:233-243

[67] Zanon MSA, Barros GG, Chulze SN. Non-aflatoxigenic *Aspergillus flavus* as potential biocontrol agents to reduce aflatoxin contamination in peanuts harvested in Northern Argentina. International Journal of Food Microbiology. 2016;**231**:63-68

[68] Peles F, Sipos P, Kovács S, Gyori Z, Pócsi I, Pusztahelyi T. Biological control and mitigation of aflatoxin contamination in commodities. Toxins. 2021;**13**:104

[69] Mostafa AA, Al-Rahmah AN, Abdel-Megeed A, Sayed SR, Hatamleh AA. Antagonistic activities of some fungal strains against the toxigenic *Aspergillus flavus* isolate and its aflatoxins productivity. Journal of Pure and Applied Microbiology. 2013;7:169-178

[70] Serrano R, Gonzalez-Menendez V, Rodríguez L, Martín J, Tormo Jrand Genilloud O. Co-culturing of fungal strains against *Botrytis cinerea* as a model for the induction of chemical diversity and therapeutic agents. Frontiers in Microbiology. 19 Apr 2017;**8**:649

[71] Kusumaningtyas E, Widiastuti Rand Maryam R. Reduction of aflatoxin B1 in chicken feed by using *Saccharomyces cerevisiae*, *Rhizopus oligosporus* and their combination. Mycopathologia. 2006;**4**:307

[72] Zhang L, Ma Q, Ma S, Zhang J, Jia R, Ji C. Ameliorating effects of Bacillus subtilis ANSB060 on growth performance, antioxidant functions, and aflatoxin residues in ducks fed diets contaminated with aflatoxins. Toxins. 2016;**1**:1

[73] Guo Y, Zhang Y, Wei C, Ma Q, Ji C, Zhang J. Efficacy of Bacillus subtilis ANSB060 biodegradation product for the reduction of the milk aflatoxin M1 content of dairy cows exposed to aflatoxin B1. Toxins. 2019;**3**:161

[74] Fan Y, Zhao L, Ji C, Li X, Jia R, Xi L. Protective effects of Bacillus subtilis ANSB060 on serum biochemistry, histopathological changes and antioxidant enzyme activities of broilers fed moldy peanut meal naturally contaminated with aflatoxins. Toxins. 2015;**8**:3330-3343

[75] Shi C, Knochel S. Susceptibility of dairy associated molds towards microbial metabolites with focus on the response to diacetyl. Food Control. Mar 2021;**121**:107573

[76] Shadjou R, Hasanzadeh M, Heidar Oor M, Shadjou N. Electrochemical monitoring of aflatoxin M1 in milk samples using silver nanoparticles dispersed on -cyclodextrin-GQDs

nanocomposite. Journal of Molecular Recognition. 2018;**31**:2699

[77] Abbas HK, Shier W, Horn B, Weaver MA. Cultural methods for aflatoxin detection. Toxicology Toxin Reviews. 2004;**23**:295-315

[78] Roman BE, Driksna D, Abouzied MM, Klein F, Rice J. Validation of MAX aqueous extraction on Veratox® for total aflatoxin ELISA test kit. AOAC International. 2017;**100**:1131-1133

[79] Sharma A, Pillai M, Gautam S, Hajare S. Mycotoxins immunological techniques for detection and analysis. In: Encyclopedia of Food Microbiology. Vol. 132. Amsterdam, The Netherlands: Elsevier; 2014. pp. 869-879

[80] Chauhan R, Solanki PR, Singh J, Mukherjee I, Basu T, Malhotra B. A novel electrochemical piezoelectric label free immunosensor for aflatoxin B1 detection in groundnut. Food Control. 2015;**52**:60-70

[81] Wacoo AP, Wendiro D, Vuzi PC, Hawumba JF. Methods for detection of aflatoxins in agricultural food crops. Applied Chemistry. 2014;**2014**(1):706291

[82] Bhardwaj H, Sumana G, Marquette CA. A label-free ultrasensitive microfluidic surface plasmon resonance biosensor for aflatoxin B1 detection using nanoparticles integrated gold chip. Food Chemistry. 2020;**307**:125530

[83] Abbas M. Chromatographic techniques for estimation of aflatoxins in food commodities. In: Aflatoxins. London, UK, London UK: Intech Open; 2021

[84] Chavez RA, Cheng X, Stasiewicz MJ. A review of the methodology of analysing aflatoxin and fumonisin in single corn kernels and the potential impacts of these methods on food security. Food. 2020;**9**:297

[85] Waliyar F, Ba A, Hassan H, Bonkoubgou S, Bose JP. Sources of resistance to *Aspergillus flavus* and aflatoxin contamination in groundnut genotypes in West Africa. Plant Diseases. 1992;**78**:704-708

[86] Pandey MK, Monyo E, Ozias-Akins P, Liang X, Guimarães P, Nigam SN, et al. Advances in arachis genomics for peanut improvement. Biotechnological Advances. 2012;**30**:639-651

[87] Pandey MK, Roorkiwal M, Singh VK, Ramalingam A, Kudapa H, Thudi M, et al. Emerging genomic tools for legume reeding: Current status and future prospects. Frontiers in Plant Sciences. 2016;**7**:455

[88] Bedre R, Rajasekaran K, Mangu VR, Timm LE, Bhatnagar D, Baisakh N. Genome-wide transcriptome analysis of cotton (*Gossypium hirsutum* L.) identifies candidate gene signatures in response to aflatoxin producing fungus *Aspergillus flavus*. PLoS One. 2015;**14**:0138025

[89] Wang H, Lei Y, Yan L, Cheng K, Dai X, Wan L, et al. Deep sequencing analysis of transcriptomes in *Aspergillus flavus* in response to resveratrol. BMC Microbiology. 2015;**15**:182

[90] Majumdar R, Lebar M, Mack B, Minocha R, Minocha S, Carter-Wientjes C, et al. The *Aspergillus flavus* spermidine synthase (spds) gene, is required for normal development, aflatoxin production, and pathogenesis during infection of maize kernels. Frontiers Plant Sciences. 2018;**9**:317

[91] Chen ZY, Brown RL, Damann KE, Cleveland TE. Identification of unique or elevated levels of Kernel proteins in aflatoxin-resistant maize

genotypes through proteome analysis. Phytopatholgia. 2002;**92**:1084-1094

[92] Brown RL, Chen ZY, Warburton M, Luo M, Menkir A, Fakhoury A, et al. Discovery and characterization of proteins associated with aflatoxin-resistance: Evaluating their potential as breeding markers. Toxins. 2010;**2**:919-933

[93] Wang T, Zhang E, Chen X, Li L, Liang X. Identification of seed proteins associated with resistance to pre-harvested aflatoxin contamination in peanut (*Arachis hypogaea* L). BMC Plant Biology. 2010;**10**:267

[94] Thakare D, Zhang J, Wing RA, Cotty PJ, Schmidt MA. Aflatoxin-free transgenic maize using host-induced gene silencing. Science Advances. 2017;**3**:e1602382

[95] Sharma KK, Pothana A, Prasad K, Shah D, Kaur J, Bhatnagar D, et al. Peanuts that keep aflatoxin at bay: A threshold that matters. Plant Biotechnology. 2018;**16**:1024-1033

[96] Adelere A, Lateef A. A novel approach to the green synthesis of metallic nanoparticles: The use of agro-wastes, enzymes, and pigments. Nanotechnological Reviews. 2016;**5**:567-587

[97] He L, Liu Y, Mustapha A, Lin MS. Antifungal activity of zinc oxide nanoparticles against *Botrytis cinerea* and *Penicillium expansum*. Microbiological Research. 2011;**166**:207-215

[98] Pietrzak K, Twaruzek M, Czyzowska A, Kosicki R, Gutarowska B. Influence of silver nanoparticles on metabolism and toxicity of moulds. Acta Biochimica Polonica. 2015;**62**:851-857

[99] Gibson N, Shenderova O, Luo TJM, Moseenkov S, Bondar V, Puzyr A, et al. Colloidal stability of modified nanodiamond particles. Diamond and Related Materials. 2009;**18**:620-626

[100] Kovac T, Sarkanj B, Klapec T, Borisev I, Kovac M, Nevistic A, et al. Fullerol $C_{60}(OH)_{24}$ nanoparticles and mycotoxigenic fungi: A preliminary investigation into modulation of mycotoxin production. Environmental Science and Pollution Research. 2017;**24**:16673-16681

[101] Puzyr AP, Purtov KV, Shenderova OA, Luo M, Brenner DW, Bondar VS. The adsorption of aflatoxin B1 by detonation-synthesis nanodiamonds. Doklady Biochemistry and Biophysics. 2007;**417**:299-301

[102] Pirouz AA, Selamat J, Iqbal SZ, Mirhosseini H, Karjiban RA, Bakar FA. The use of innovative and efficient nanocomposite (magnetic graphene oxide) for the reduction on of fusarium mycotoxins in palm kernel cake. Scientific Reports. 2017;**7**:12453

[103] Khajarern JM, Khajarern S, Moon TH, Lee JH. Effects of dietary supplementation of fermented chitin-chitosan (fermkit) on toxicity of mycotoxin in ducks. Asian-Australasian Journal of Animal Sciences. 2003;**16**:706-713

[104] Zhao Z, Liu N, Yang L, Wang J, Song S, Nie D, et al. Cross-linked chitosan polymers as generic adsorbents for simultaneous adsorption of multiple mycotoxins. Food Control. 2015;**57**:362-369

[105] Skalickova S, Milosavljevic V, Cihalova K, Horky P, Richtera L, Adam V. Selenium nanoparticles as a nutritional supplement. Nutrition. 2017;**33**:83-90

[106] Kovacic P, Somanathan R. Biomechanisms of nanoparticles

(toxicants, antioxidants and therapeutics): Electron transfer and reactive oxygen species. Nanoscience and Nanotechnology. 2010;**10**:7919-7930

[107] Nelson BC, Johnson ME, Walker ML, Riley KR, Sims CM. Antioxidant cerium oxide nanoparticles in biology and medicine. Antioxidants. 2016;**5**:15

[108] Navale GR, Thripuranthaka M, Late DJ, Shinde SS. Antimicrobial activity of ZnO nanoparticles against pathogenic bacteria and fungi. JSM Nanotechnology and Nanomedicine. 2015;**3**(1):1033

[109] Kanhed P, Birla S, Gaikwad S, Gade A, Seabra AB, Rubilar O, et al. In vitro antifungal efficacy of copper nanoparticles against selected crop pathogenic fungi. Materials Letters. 2014;**115**:13-17

[110] Abdel-Hadi AM, Awad MF, Abo-Dahab NF, ElKady MF. Extracellular synthesis of silver nanoparticles by *Aspergillus terreus*: Biosynthesis, characterization and biological activity. Biosciences Biotechnology Research Asia. 2014;**11**(3):1179-1186

[111] Mukherjee K, Acharya K, Biswas A, Jana NR. TiO_2 nanoparticles co doped with nitrogen and fluorine as visible-light activated antifungal agents. ACS Applied Nano Materials. 2020;**3**(2):2016-2025

[112] Sun S, Zhao R, Xie Y, Liu Y. Photocatalytic degradation of aflatoxin B_1 by activated carbon supported TiO_2 catalyst. Food Control. 2019;**100**:183-188

[113] Bai X, Sun C, Liu D, Luo X, Li D, Wang J, et al. Photocatalytic degradation of deoxynivalenol using graphene/ZnO hybrids in aqueous suspension. Applied Catalysis B: Environmental. 2017;**204**:11-20

[114] Wu C, He J, Li Y, Chen N, Huang Z, You L, et al. Solid phase extraction of aflatoxins using a nanosorbent consisting of amagnetized nanoporous carbon core coated with a molecularly imprinted polymer. Microchimica Acta. 2018;**185**(11):515

[115] Devipriya D, Roopan SM. *Cissus quadrangularis* mediated ecofriendly synthesis of copper oxide nanoparticles and its antifungal studies against *Aspergillus niger*, *Aspergillus flavus*. Materials of Science and Engineering C Materials of Applied Bioscience. 2017;**80**:38-44

[116] Shakibaie M, Mohazab NS, Mousavi SAA. Antifungal activity of selenium nanoparticles synthesized by bacillus species Msh-1 against *Aspergillus fumigatus* and *Candida albicans*. Microbiology. 2015;**8**:e26381

[117] Madbouly AK, Abdel-Aziz MS, Abdel-Wahhab MA. Biosynthesis of nanosilver using *Chaetomium globosum* and its application to control *Fusarium* wilt of tomato in the greenhouse. IET Nanobiotechnology. 2017;**11**:702-708

[118] Medda S, Hajra A, Dey U, Bose P, Mondal NK. Biosynthesis of silver nanoparticles from *Aloe vera* leaf extract and antifungal activity against *Rhizopus* sp. and *Aspergillus* sp. Applied Nanosciences. 2015;**5**:875-880

[119] Yassin MA, El-Samawaty AMA, Dawoud TM, Abd-Elkader OH, Al Maary KS, Hatamleh AA, et al. Characterization and anti-*Aspergillus flavus* impact of nanoparticles synthesized by *Penicillium citrinum*. Biological Sciences. 2017;**24**:1243-1248

[120] Xue BJ, He D, Gao S, Wang DY, Yokoyama K, Wang L. Biosynthesis of silver nanoparticles by the fungus *Arthroderma fulvum* and its antifungal

activity against genera of *Candida*, *aspergillus* and *Fusarium*. Nanomedicine. 2016;**11**:1899-1906

[121] Ammar HAM, El-Desouky TA. Green synthesis of nanosilver particles by aspergillus terreus HA1N and *Penicillium expansum* HA2N and its antifungal activity against mycotoxigenic fungi. Applied Microbiology. 2016;**121**:89-100

[122] Mao J, Zhang Q, Li P, Zhang L, Zhang W. Geometric architecture design of ternary composites based on dispersive WO_3 nanowires for enhanced visible light-driven activity of refractory pollutant degradation. Chemical Engineering Journal. 2018;**334**:2568-2578

[123] Karami-Osboo R, Mirabolfathi M. A novel dispersive nanomagnetic particle solid-phase extraction method to determine aflatoxins in nut and cereal samples. Food Analytical Methods. 2017;**10**(12):4086-4093

[124] Zhang X, Li G, Wu D, Yu Y, Hu N, Wang H, et al. Emerging strategies for the activity assay and inhibitor screening of alpha-glucosidase. Food & Function. 2020;**11**(1):66-82

[125] Chen C, Yu X, Han D, Ai J, Ke Y, Wang Z, et al. Non- CTAB synthesized gold nanorods-based immunochromatographic assay for dual color and on-site detection of aflatoxins and zearalenones in maize. Food Control. 2020;*118*:107418

[126] Xue Z, Zhang Y, Yu W, Zhang J, Wang J, Wan F, et al. Recent advances in aflatoxin B1 detection based on nanotechnology and nanomaterials-a review. Analytica Chimica Acta. 2019;**1069**:1-27

[127] Goud KY, Kailasa SK, Kumar V, Tsang YF, Gobi KV, Kim KH. Progress on nanostructured electrochemical sensors and their recognition elements for detection of mycotoxins. A Review of Biosensors and Bioelectronics. 2018;**121**:205-222

[128] Zhang X, Li G, Wu D, Li X, Hu N, Chen J, et al. Recent progress in the design fabrication of metal-organic frameworks-based nanozymes and their applications to sensing and cancer therapy. Biosensors and Bioelectronics. 2019;**137**:178-198

[129] Tian F, Zhou J, Jiao B, He Y. A nanozyme-based cascade colorimetric aptasensor for amplified detection of ochratoxin A. Nanoscale. 2019;**11**(19):9547-9555

[130] Yang X, Qian J, Jiang L, Yan Y, Wang K, Liu Q, et al. Ultrasensitive electrochemical aptasensor for ochratoxin A based on two level cascaded signal amplification strategy. Bioelectrochemistry. 2014;**96**:7-13

[131] Taghdisi SM, Danesh NM, Beheshti HR, Ramezani M, Abnous K. A novel fluorescent aptasensor based on gold and silica nanoparticles for the ultrasensitive detection of ochratoxin A. Nanoscale. 2016;**8**(6):3439-3446

[132] Chatterjee B, Das SJ, Anand A, Sharma TK. Nanozymes and aptamer-based biosensing. Materials Science for Energy Technologies. 2020;**3**:127-135

[133] Sun S, Zhao R, Feng S, Xie Y. Colorimetric zearalenone assay based on the use of an aptamer and of gold nanoparticles with peroxidase-like activity. Microchimica Acta. 2018;**185**(12):535

[134] Huang L, Chen K, Zhang W, Zhu W, Liu X, Wang J. ssDNA-tailorable oxidase-mimicking activity of spinel $MnCo_2O_4$ for sensitive biomolecular detection in

food sample. Sensors and Actuators B-Chemical. 2018;**269**:79-87

[135] Zhu W, Li L, Zhou Z, Yang X, Hao N, Guo Y, et al. A colorimetric biosensor for simultaneous ochratoxin A and aflatoxins B1 detection in agricultural products. Food Chemistry. 2020;**319**:126544

[136] Mitra C, Gummadidala PM, Afshinnia K, Merrifield RC, Baalousha M, Lead JR, et al. Citrate-coated silver nanoparticles growth-independently inhibit synthesis in aspergillus parasiticus. Environmental Science and Technology. 2017;**51**:8085-8093

[137] Mousavi SAA, Pourtalebi S. Inhibitory effects of silver nanoparticles on growth and aflatoxin B-1 production by *Aspergillus parasiticus*. Medical Science. 2015;**40**:501-506

[138] Rashed AM, Mohamed A-EAAR, Abobakr MM. Wheat protection from root rot caused by *Fusarium culmorum* using silver nanoparticles. Chemical Society of Pakistan. 2016;**38**:898-903

[139] Kheiri A, Moosawi Jorf SA, Malihipour A, Saremi H, Nikkhah M. Synthesis and characterization of chitosan nanoparticles and their effect on fusarium head blight and oxidative activity in wheat. Biological Macromolecules. 2017;**102**:526-538

[140] Dananjaya HS, Erandani W, Kim CH, Nikapitiya C, Lee J, De Zoysa M. Comparative study on antifungal activities of chitosan nanoparticles and chitosan silver nanocomposites against *Fusarium oxysporum* species complex. Biological Macromolecules. 2017;**105**:478-488

[141] Shenashen M, Derbalah A, Hamza A, Mohamed A, El Safty S. Antifungal activity of fabricated mesoporous alumina nanoparticles against root rot disease of tomato caused by *Fusarium oxysporium*. Pest Management Science. 2017;**73**:1121-1126

[142] Solanki PR, Singh J, Rupavali B, Tiwari S, Malhotra BD. Bismuth oxide nanorods based immunosensor for mycotoxin detection. Materials of Science and Engineering C Materials of Applied Biology. 2017;**70**:564-571

[143] Zeng XL, Zhang FQ, He NY, Zhang BY, Liu XY, Li XL. ZnO nanoparticles of different shapes and their antimycotic property against penicillium and mucor. Nanoscience and Nanotechnology Letters. 2016;**8**:688-694

[144] Goryacheva IY, De Saeger S. Immunochemical detection of masked mycotoxins: A short review. World Mycotoxin. 2012;**5**:281-287

[145] Huybrechts B, Martins JC, Debongnie P, Uhlig S, Callebaut A. Fast and sensitive LC-MS/MS method measuring human mycotoxin exposure using biomarkers in urine. Archieves of Toxicology. 2015;**89**:1993-2005

[146] Nakagawa H, Ohmichi K, Sakamoto S, Sago Y, Kushiro M, Nagashima H, et al. Detection of a new Fusarium masked mycotoxin in wheat grain by high-resolution LC-Orbitrap™ MS. Food Additives & Contaminants. Part A, Chemistry, Analysis, Control, Exposure & Risk Assessment. 2011;**28**:1447-1456

[147] Niemirowicz K, Durnas B, Piktel E, Bucki R. Development of antifungal therapies using nanomaterials. Nanomedicine. 2017;**12**:1891-1905

[148] Petrakova AV, Urusov AE, Zherdev AV, Liu L, Xu C, Dzantiev BB. Application of magnetite nanoparticles for the development of highly sensitive

immunochromatographic test systems for mycotoxin detection. Applied Biochemistry and Microbiology. 2017;**53**:470-475

[149] Kong D, Liu L, Song S, Suryoprabowo S, Li A, Kuang H, et al. A goldnanoparticle-basedsemi-quantitative and quantitative ultrasensitive paper sensor for the detection of twenty mycotoxins. Nanoscale. 2016;**8**:5245-5253

[150] Aqai P, Peters J, Gerssen A, HaasnootW, NielenWF. Immunomagnetic microbeads for screening with flow cytometry and identification with nano-liquid chromatography mass spectrometry of ochratoxins in wheat and cereal. Analytical Bioanalytical Chemistry. 2011;**400**:3085-3096

[151] Roque L, Molpeceres J, Reis C, Rijo P, Reis CP. Past recent progresses and future perspectives of nanotechnology applied to antifungal agents. Current Drug Metabolism. 2017;**18**:280-290

[152] Majumder S, Shakil NA, Kumar J, Banerjee T, Sinha P, Singh BB, et al. Eco-friendly peg-based controlled release nano-formulations of Mancozeb: Synthesis and bioefficacy evaluation against phytopathogenic fungi *Alternaria solani* and *Sclerotium rolfsii*. Journal of Environmental Science and Health - Part B Pesticides, Food Contaminants, and Agricultural Wastes. 2016;**51**:873-880

[153] Khalili ST, Mohsenifar A, Beyki M, Zhaveh S, Rahmani-Cherati T, Abdollahi A, et al. Encapsulation of thyme essential oils in chitosan-benzoic acid nanogel with enhanced antimicrobial activity against *Aspergillus flavus*. LWT-Food Science and Technology. 2015;**60**:502-508

[154] Zhaveh S, Mohsenifar A, Beiki M, Khalili ST, Abdollahi A, Rahmani-Cherati T, et al. Encapsulation of *Cuminum cyminum* essential oils in chitosan-caffeic acid nanogel with enhanced antimicrobial activity against *Aspergillus flavus*. Industrial Crops and Products. 2015;**69**:251-256

[155] Li HB, Shen QS, Zhou W, Mo HZ, Pan DD, Hu LB. Nanocapsular dispersion of cinnamaldehyde for enhanced inhibitory activity against aflatoxin production by *Aspergillus flavus*. Molecules. 2015;**20**:6022-6032

[156] Zhao J, Wang L, Xu D, Lu ZS. Involvement of ROS in nanosilver-caused suppression of aflatoxin production from *Aspergillus flavus*. RSC Advances. 2017;**7**:23021-23026

[157] Yu KP, Huang YT, Yang SC. The antifungal efficacy of nano-metals supported TiO_2 and ozone on the resistant *Aspergillus Niger* spore. Hazardous Material. 2013;**261**:155-162

[158] Pinto JB, Almeida A, Fernandes SCM, Freire CSR, Silvestre AJD, Neto CP, et al. Antifungal activity of transparent nanocomposite thin films of pullulan and silver against *Aspergillus Niger*. Colloids and Surfaces B Biointerfaces. 2013;**103**:143-148

Chapter 5

Aflatoxins in Staple Foods in Latin America and the Caribbean Countries and Decontamination Strategies

Donna M. Morrison, Ram K. Shrestha and Andréia Bianchini

Abstract

Cassava, maize, and rice are the main staple foods of Latin America and the Caribbean (LAC) region, and these crops are highly susceptible to fungal contamination and the metabolites of fungi, including aflatoxins. The presence of aflatoxins in foods is a serious risk to human health, causing acute and chronic effects. They are produced at all production, storage, and marketing stages of crops and their by-products when conditions for handling and storage are not well managed. This chapter provides a comprehensive overview of aflatoxins in cassava, maize, and rice in the Latin America and the Caribbean region and mitigation strategies. It also outlines the potential impact on food security in the region. The findings showed that aflatoxins are prevalent across Latin America and the Caribbean countries. Despite the application of mitigation strategies, there are still concerns about risks to human health due to the high consumption of staple foods. Hence, governmental and institutional interventions are essential to developing sustainable strategies that prevent food contamination and protect public health in the region.

Keywords: aflatoxins, cassava, maize, rice, processing, decontamination

1. Introduction

The Latin America and the Caribbean region is diverse in background and culture, comprising three main areas: continental South America, Central America, and the Caribbean. South America comprises thirteen countries, while Central America includes seven countries. The Caribbean was named after the islands' original inhabitants, The Carib. The Caribbean Islands are divided into three major subdivisions. The Bahamas are a grouping of flat islands in the northern reaches of the Caribbean archipelago; the Greater Antilles are large islands in the western Caribbean; and the Lesser Antilles are smaller islands in the eastern Caribbean that form a crescent between Puerto Rico and Venezuela [1]. The tapestry of Latin America and the Caribbean is woven by a history of colonizers, slavery, indentured laborers, and immigration. This has impacted culture, language, and identity. Following the conquest of the indigenous people in the region, most countries adopted the languages of the colonizers—English, French, Spanish, and Portuguese. Suriname is the only country where the national language is Dutch. Areas with Indigenous populations in most countries still use their native languages.

Latin American and Caribbean cuisine is a rich fusion of indigenous traditions, colonial influences, and culinary contributions from Africans, Asians, and Europeans. The main staple foods produced and consumed throughout most of Latin America and the Caribbean are maize, rice, cassava (yucca), beans, and milk. In Latin America, more than half of the diet comprises carbohydrates from grains, pasta, and bread [2]. Rice, cassava, and maize are highly susceptible to fungal contamination at both pre-harvest and post-harvest stages, including distribution and marketing. This chapter focuses on the methods applicable to control post-harvest contamination of aflatoxins in cassava, maize, and rice, as well as during the processing of these selected crops.

2. Staple foods in Latin America and the Caribbean and food security

Cassava, maize, and rice are Latin America and the Caribbean three major staple food crops. These crops represent the foundation of daily diets and are important foods for the region to achieve the United Nations Sustainable Development Goals. Nutritionally, these crops are rich in carbohydrates, acting as a vital energy source while offering essential protein, vitamins, and minerals to support the population's overall health. However, in the case of maize, fortification is needed to enhance nutrition [3].

Latin America and the Caribbean achieved the Millennium Development Goals (MDGs) for halving the proportion of people suffering from hunger between 1990 and 2015. However, since then, there has been an increase in the number of people facing hunger and food insecurity. In 2022, 38% of the region's population suffered from food insecurity (247.8 million people), and 7% (43 million) faced hunger [4]. Focusing on the four pillars of food security (physical availability of food, economic and physical access to food, food utilization and stability), the recommendations of the Inter-American Development Bank are to adapt agricultural policies to increase the availability of nutritious and healthy foods; identify and protect the most vulnerable people from food insecurity; generate nutrition-sensitive agricultural interventions that promote the production and consumption of nutritious foods; and promote shorter supply chains that encourage local production and consumption [4]. To this end, rural farmers should be given access to resources and knowledge of modern technology applied to crop production. Governments and various agencies should be integrally involved in investments to promote rural development and reduce migration to urban communities. In addition, there must be a network of roads and transportation to allow the distribution of produce and other crops from rural farmers to urban communities and access to facilities that promote international export. Clear policies should focus on driving the productivity of indigenous crops to provide affordable food for local consumers and increase competitiveness. In 2022, the proportion of the population unable to afford a healthy diet in the Caribbean and Latin America was 50% and 26.1%, respectively, compared to 35.4% globally [5]. Of greater significance is that the Caribbean countries import between 32.4% and 96.2% of their staple foods [6]. Therefore, Latin America and the Caribbean should rethink agriculture and retool farmers with skills to improve efficiency and quality. This will help them maximize profits, and in the long term, it should lower the food import bill in these countries.

The United Nations' objectives of food security also encapsulate access to safe foods [7]. Therefore, as a region, equal attention should also be focused on food safety. Unsafe food poses serious health risks, particularly to infants, young children, the elderly, and immunocompromised individuals, increasing their vulnerability to disease [8]. Overall, contamination of food reduces availability and threatens human and animal health and livelihoods. Hence, all members of the production and marketing chain should be trained in food safety and the methods of producing safe foods.

2.1 Aflatoxins

Mycotoxins are naturally occurring chemical contaminants in food and feed that pose significant risks to human and animal health. These are secondary metabolites produced by various fungal species at different stages of crop production and throughout the food chain. There are over 300 mycotoxins and emerging mycotoxins globally [9, 10]. The most important classes are aflatoxins, trichothecenes, fumonisins, ochratoxin A, and zearalenone. Aflatoxins are a group 1 carcinogen since there is evidence that they cause hepatocellular carcinoma (HCC) in humans [11]. The four major types of aflatoxins are AFB_1, AFB_2, AFG_1, and AFG_2, of which AFB_1 is the most potent. Due to their high heat resistance and high decomposition temperatures, aflatoxins remain a significant risk in food products [12]. Human exposure primarily occurs through contaminated food. Aflatoxins are produced by the fungi *Aspergillus* section *Flavi*, present in hot, humid climates, and *Aspergillus parasiticus*, adapted to the soil environment. Contamination by aflatoxin-producing fungi during production may occur at early stages of crop development and is influenced by dry, hot conditions. In contrast, at later stages, when the crop is matured, it is affected by warm, wet conditions. Rainfall and contamination at later stages are directly correlated [13]. Hence, Latin America and the Caribbean climate is suitable for the growth and infestation of crops by microorganisms, including aflatoxigenic fungi, and the production of aflatoxins.

2.2 Toxicity of aflatoxins to human health

Intake of foods contaminated with aflatoxin constitutes a serious public health risk, including increased chances of liver cancer, immune system suppression, and stunted growth in children [14]. Human exposure to aflatoxin primarily occurs through the consumption of food contaminated with *Aspergillus flavus* or *A. parasiticus* and their secondary metabolites [15, 16]. For example, it was observed that there is a direct association between the consumption of tortillas made from maize masa and the AFB_1-lys concentration in human blood [17]. Aflatoxin B_1, the most toxic form of aflatoxin, significantly increases the risk of HCC, a primary form of liver cancer [11]. Large doses of aflatoxins lead to acute illness and death, and chronic or sublethal doses resulting from exposure to relatively low concentrations over an extended period have nutritional and immunological consequences. The cumulative effect of all doses directly correlates with the risk of cancer [18, 19]. The risk for carcinogenicity is greater in developing countries with a less varied diet and possibly lower quality foods, such as those in Latin America and the Caribbean than in developed countries with more varied diets [20]. Diet may contribute to the high incidence of HCC in Guatemala, where maize, a cereal highly susceptible to aflatoxigenic fungi and other fungi, is responsible for a significant portion of the daily diet [21, 22]. An investigation in Guatemala found that all subjects had significant levels of AFB_1-lysine in their blood, indicative of their risk for liver cancer. Rural and Indigenous Guatemalans had the highest exposure, with the Indigenous and rural males having the highest AFB1-lys adduct compared to other studied groups [23]. In Brazil, it was determined that lactating women are exposed to potentially dangerous levels of aflatoxins in the foods they consume, mainly maize and maize products, resulting in a high risk for HCC [24]. There have been a few cases of acute aflatoxicosis in humans. One such case occurred in Kenya, where in 2004, several hundred Kenyans became severely ill, and 125 died of acute aflatoxicosis. Aflatoxin-linked liver cancer is the most common liver disease in Sub-Saharan Africa and in the world [25, 26].

Apart from HCC, there are other symptoms of aflatoxicosis. These include hemorrhagic necrosis of the liver, bile duct proliferation, edema, and lethargy [27]. In 2006, Brazil had an outbreak of the disease beri beri, resulting in some fatalities. It was suggested that this may have been due to aflatoxins associated with poor rice storage [28]. Consumption of maize with aflatoxin is responsible for stunted growth and intestinal dysbiosis in children of Guatemala [29]. The direct association between the high aflatoxin concentration in the breast milk of lactating mothers and the aflatoxin concentration in infants' urine may explain the observed stunted growth [30]. It was also determined that there is an increased risk of lung cancer for persons exposed to dusty conditions in rice mills [31]. Cytotoxicity and apoptosis occur in the lungs because of affected respiratory reactive centers [32].

2.3 Regulatory limits for aflatoxins in foods

Mycotoxin regulatory limits on food and feed are critical in protecting public health. Such limits are established by institutions and individual countries' standards organizations to monitor and control the public health risks associated with consuming mycotoxins. The regulatory limits for aflatoxins somewhat vary across countries and institutions in Latin America and the Caribbean. For example, in South America, Argentina recommends a maximum residual limit (MRL) of 20 μg/kg in all foods, while for Peru, it is 10 μg/kg. The Mercosur countries (full members—Argentina, Brazil, Bolivia, Paraguay, and Uruguay, along with seven associate members) have established MRLs for total AFLs ($AFB_1 + AFB_2 + AFG_1 + AFG_2$) of 20 μg/Kg for products that contain peanut and maize. In the Caribbean, Barbados' requirement for all foods is 20 μg/Kg. Guatemala's recommendation for specific foods, including maize and rice, is 20 μg/Kg [33, 34]. Regarding maize, standards ranging from 4 μg/Kg to 20 μg/Kg should provide some level of protection from aflatoxins if the objective is 1 in 10,000 lifetime HCC, except in cases where there is a high consumption [35].

2.4 Economic losses due to the presence of aflatoxins in staple foods of Latin and the Caribbean

There are limited studies on the economic losses due to aflatoxins in foods in Latin America and the Caribbean. Given the susceptibility of staple foods to aflatoxins, there is the potential for financial losses at all stages of the production and marketing chain if good agricultural practices and efficient post-harvest management strategies are not applied. The farmers may have to discard damaged crops, decreasing the available supply for consumers and representing a loss of revenue for the farmers. Deficiencies in conditions during storage, distribution, and handling would result in the loss of crops and consequent depression of profits. Farmers, exporters, and distributors may also incur costs for testing their products to determine the extent of contamination caused by mycotoxins. If there is a likelihood that the products are contaminated with aflatoxins, importers may decline to buy the product or may offer lower prices, resulting in a loss of revenue [36, 37]. Such actions can hurt the economies of the exporting countries, significantly impacting lower- and middle-income countries.

The consumption of food with aflatoxin may lead to illnesses and deaths that can be an economic burden to society due to the cost of health care and reduction in human capital stock measured as disability-adjusted life years due to years of life lost to premature mortality and loss of years of healthy life due to disability [27]. The symptoms of acute illness may appear early after ingestion. In contrast, for chronic disease, the effect may be insidious in the early stages, becoming difficult to treat and recover at later stages.

3. Cassava as a staple food in Latin America and the Caribbean

Cassava, the third most important source of calories in the tropics after rice and maize, is now cultivated in over 90 countries and is a staple for half a billion people in Africa, Asia, Latin America, and the Caribbean [38]. In Latin American and Caribbean countries, cassava contributes 16% and 10.2%, respectively, of the population's diet energy supply when wheat, maize, and rice are excluded [39]. The shrubby plant *Manihot esculenta*—the scientific name for cassava—and its wild relatives of the genus *Manihot* originate in Brazil. The name cassava is theorized to be derived from the word Casavi or Cazabi in the language of the Arawak (the first indigenous people who lived in the Greater Antilles), which translates to bread. It is also known as manioc, mandioca, or yucca in South America or tapioca in Asia. It is a perennial woody shrub that may grow 1–4 m high and belongs to the dicotyledon family Euphorbiaceae. Cultivated mainly for its starchy roots, it is considered a complete food since all plant parts can be consumed [40, 41]. Indigenous peoples first domesticated the plant, and Portuguese sailors took it to Africa in the sixteenth century; from there, its use spread to tropical Asia, reaching as far as Indonesia. Every tropical country has the conditions to cultivate cassava, but most cultivation is concentrated in north and eastern Paraguay, northwestern South America, and the Greater Antilles. The crop's traits allow it to be cultivated in marginal soil and tolerate acid, drought stress, soil infertility, and defoliation by pests. Cassava has the highest yield (and carbohydrate production) per hectare than other cereal crops [42, 43]. Cassava is grown in almost every South, Meso-America, and Caribbean country. Seven countries produce 96% of the production in the Americas [44]. In the year 2022, Brazil had the highest production of cassava in Latin America and the Caribbean with over 17 million tonnes, followed by Paraguay with over 2 million tonnes, then Peru with almost 1.5 million tonnes [45], as displayed in **Table 1**.

3.1 Nutritional composition and anti-nutrients of cassava

The nutritional composition of cassava depends on the plant's geographical location, variety, age, and environmental conditions under which it is grown. There are two types of cassava—bitter and sweet. The bitter cassava has more toxins (cyanogenic glycosides) than the sweet, and many local varieties exist throughout the region. The root is rich in carbohydrates with a relatively smaller concentration of proteins and fiber. The carbohydrates in roots include mainly starch (amylose and

Cassava		Maize		Rice	
Country	**Production ('000 Tonnes)**	**Country**	**Production ('000 Tonnes)**	**Country**	**Production ('000 Tonnes)**
Brazil	17648.5	Brazil	109420.7	Brazil	10776.3
Paraguay	2617.9	Argentina	59037.2	Peru	3449.4
Peru	1389.8	Mexico	26625.7	Colombia	2620.1
Colombia	1019.0	Paraguay	6191.7	Uruguay	1372.7
Cuba	717.8	Guatemala	1950.0	Ecuador	1252.8
Haiti	647.3	Colombia	1921.2	Argentina	1222.4
Venezuela	378.9	Ecuador	1641.1	Dominican Republic	1149
Nicaragua	275.3	Peru	1611.8	Guyana	929.6
Bolivia	216.6	Venezuela	1352.6	Paraguay	861.5
Argentina	201.0	Bolivia	985.6	Bolivia	608.7

Source: [45].

Table 1.
The top ten highest producers of cassava, maize, and rice in Latin America and the Caribbean in 2022.

amylopectin) and small amounts of fructose, sucrose, glucose, and maltose. It is also composed of vitamins and minerals, with vitamins A (β-carotene) and C being the most predominant. Both leaves and roots have calcium, iron, potassium, magnesium, copper, zinc, and manganese. The leaves, however, have higher quantities of protein and lipids than the roots [46–48].

In contrast, there is a significant presence of anti-nutrients. These are natural or synthetic compounds that interfere with the absorption of nutrients [49]. The most consequential anti-nutrient in cassava is endogenously stored cyanogenic glycosides. These are stable compounds, but through the action of β-glycosidase, cyanohydrin is formed, which in turn dissociates to form hydrogen cyanide (HCN) [50]. The young leaves produce a higher concentration of HCN compared to the roots. Consumption of unprocessed cassava can cause acute and chronic effects. Although acute intoxication is rare, the effects of chronic intoxication include exacerbation of protein deficiency, goiter, rickets, diabetes associated with calcification of the pancreas, cancer, and congenital malformations [51]. In 2017, an incident of poisoning occurred in Kasese District, Uganda, due to the consumption of products made from cassava flour with high concentrations of cyanogenic glycosides. This resulted in 98 probable cases and two deaths [52]. Reduction of cyanide can be achieved by applying processing methods, including extrusion, dry-milling, cooking, and solid-state fermentation [53–56].

Other anti-nutrients of cassava roots and leaves include tannins, polyphenols, oxalates, nitrates, saponins, and phytates [38, 57]. Studies have demonstrated that anti-nutrients in dried leaves change with maturity. While nitrates decreased with maturity, saponin, polyphenols, and cyanide increased. Regarding human health, saponins have antioxidants, anti-tumor, hypoglycemic, hypocholesterolemic, and anti-inflammatory properties but can also be hemolytic [58, 59]. Polyphenols reduce the digestibility of proteins, while oxalates bind calcium, preventing their absorption [60]. Processing cassava is necessary to reduce anti-nutrients and improve the bioavailability of desired nutrients [61].

3.2 Cassava processing in Latin America and the Caribbean

Cassava is processed into several products. Minimal processing includes peeling, washing, cutting, sanitizing, packaging, and refrigerating the cut roots. In other forms of processing, following cleaning, the roots may be cooked by baking, frying, and steaming (boiling). Grated cassava is dried or roasted, made into flour, then formed into a savory dough to make biscuits, bread, flatbread, cakes, pasta, pastries, croquettes, dumplings, and other products. Cassava is also made into starch (a dried, white powdered product), which can serve as a thickening agent in foods such as sauces, soups, and broths. The grated pulp may also be made into farinha, a staple in Brazil, which then is used to prepare farofa, a typical Brazilian dish [44]. The leaves are consumed as a vegetable, a component in salads, or as an ingredient in relish [38, 62–64]. Casareep, made by boiling down the juice of grated cassava with added spices such as cinnamon, originated in the Indigenous communities of Guyana. Its use is now widespread to flavor sauces and meat and to make a Guyanese dish, pepperpot [65]. In Brazil, fermented cassava is used to prepare alcoholic or non-alcoholic beverages, including Tarubá and Yakupa [66].

3.3 Aflatoxins in cassava and cassava products

Cassava can become contaminated with aflatoxigenic fungi and, consequently, aflatoxins while still in the soil, during processing, handling, and storage. Cassava is cultivated for its tuberous roots, which are directly in contact with the soil. It is harvested by cutting the stem and digging out the roots using an appropriate tool. Efforts should be made to avoid damaging the roots while harvesting since the damaged areas may be entry points for fungal contamination. In preparation for further processing, the roots are peeled. This should be done with clean implements to limit contamination, and the peeled cassava should be placed in clean containers while preventing contact with the ground.

A study of *Aspergillus* section *Flavi* and aflatoxin in cassava and cassava products in Brazil found that the source of the fungus in cassava tubers was likely the soil. *Aspergillus flavus* had the highest frequency of occurrence in the root, while *Aspergillus parasiticus* had the highest number of isolates from the soil. *Aspergillus arachidicola and Aspergillus novoparasiticus* were also isolated from the soil and tubers. Aflatoxins were not present in the cassava tubers [67]. Other investigations on cassava tubers showed similar results. After further observations, it was proposed that at this stage, the root may be resistant to the formation of aflatoxin or cyanide in the cassava tubers, which may prevent fungal secondary metabolism [68, 69].

Storage and packing conditions can significantly impact the overall quality of cassava products. Cassava products with high moisture content showed increased mold growth during drying, with a positive correlation between storage duration and aflatoxin concentration. The longer the drying period, the more exposure leading to mold and insect infestation. In addition, drying cassava in the open on bare soil, on tarpaulin, or on paved ground further exacerbates the problem [70]. A direct relationship between storage time and aflatoxin concentration was also observed in both fermented and unfermented cassava products, especially when stored in plastic bags that were then placed in jute bags [71]. In Uganda, cassava chips and flour are packaged in plastic single-layered gunny bags, and the majority of farmers (86.7%) store the products on the ground in the family house and not in separate rooms on pallets that are slightly above the ground [72]. The Ugandan researchers point to the need for all members of the cassava value chain to become knowledgeable about mycotoxin and trained in preventative methods. Implementing good manufacturing practices(GMPs) ensures the production of high-quality, aflatoxin-free cassava flour [73].

Studies on cassava products showed varying results depending on the production process. In Brazil, cassava starch/cassava gum and sour starch had no AFB_1, while cassava flour had traces of AFB_1 [57, 74]. In Guyana, a study on cassava meal, that is prepared similar to that of cassava flour, and cassava bread yielded no detectable aflatoxin [75]. During the production of cassava flour, after peeling and cleaning, the dried roots/chips are soaked in water for 12–16 hours, leading to fermentation and the emergence of lactic acid bacteria and *Saccharomyces cerevisiae* that can bind or degrade aflatoxin [76–78]. This might be one of the reasons for the non-detection of aflatoxins in cassava flour produced in Tanzania [79]. A study focused on three Indigenous populations of the Colombian Amazon detected no aflatoxin in cassava processed by fermenting for three days, followed by drying for two days, then roasting [80]. Similarly, cassava chips may become contaminated with fungus, including aflatoxigenic fungi, but have no aflatoxins [68, 81].

Overall, it can be concluded that cassava and cassava products can become contaminated with fungus where moisture content is conducive to their growth and development. Thermal processes remove the moisture, leaving the products dry and prohibiting fungal growth. In addition, other methods, such as fermentation, may degrade the mycotoxin.

4. Maize as a staple food in Latin America and the Caribbean

Maize (*Zea mays* L. subsp. mays), also known as corn, is the second most cultivated crop in the world and, together with rice and wheat, is one of the three major cereal crops. It is the primary staple of Latin America and the Caribbean, where it is cultivated on 10 million hectares, producing about 30 million tonnes annually [82]. Maize was first domesticated in Mexico in about 7000 B.C. Culture, ethnogeography, anthropology, and history shaped maize migration to Latin America and the Caribbean. Evidence from the Dominican Republic, Cuba, and Saba showed that maize was being consistently exploited as early as 3000 B.C. up to the "contact period" around 1500 A.D. Maize has influenced cuisines, rites, and rituals of Latin America and the Caribbean [83–85]. The importance of maize as a staple in Latin America and the Caribbean region is reflected in its increased production, which was 56.7 million tonnes in 1990–1992 and is projected to reach 135.2 million tonnes in 2030 [86]. In the year 2022, Brazil had the highest production of maize in Latin America and the Caribbean region with over 109 million tonnes, followed by Argentina (>59 million tonnes), then Mexico (>26 million tonnes) [45] as shown in **Table 1**. Brazil has become the leading producer and exporter of maize in Latin America and the Caribbean region, achieved by improvements in crop production, new seeds (both hybrid and genetically modified), and expansion into new territories. In addition, Brazil and Argentina have adopted the no-till method of cultivation, which accounts for a significant increase in yield [87].

4.1 Nutritional composition of maize

Maize is a nutritionally significant crop primarily providing macronutrients, including carbohydrates, protein, and fat, while it also offers a range of micronutrients, including vitamins and minerals. The dried maize grains generally contain more than 70% starch, approximately 6.8 to 12.0% protein, 12.0%water, 3.4% fat, and 1% ash and crude fibers. Maize is rich in high-sulfur proteins and the amino acids methionine and cysteine; however, it is deficient in some essential amino acids, including lysine and tryptophan. In addition to vitamin A, maize contains important B vitamins, including niacin (B_3), biotin (B_7), thiamin (B_1), and pyridoxine (B_6). Additionally, it also contains folic acid, potassium, selenium, and phytochemicals [88, 89].

4.2 Maize processing in Latin America and the Caribbean

Raw maize undergoes various processing methods before transforming into food for human consumption. Nixtamalization is a widely accepted maize processing method that has been adopted throughout Latin America and the Caribbean region. It improves maize's nutritional value, as well as its culinary and sensory attributes. Nixtamalization involves soaking or cooking kernels in an alkaline solution that originally was mainly made using wood ash (potassium hydroxide). This solution is now prepared with lime (calcium hydroxide) or other calcium salts. The kernels are cooked in the lime (alkaline solution) for about 1 hour and are left to steep overnight. The liquor is discarded, and the cooked kernels are rinsed to remove the lime. The softened maize is ground to form "masa," which is then used to prepare dough to make tortillas [90], or other products as outlined in **Figure 1**. During the process, solubilization of the outer pericarp occurs, followed by its removal, facilitating easier processing of the kernel into flour and masa. Nixtamalization also increases the availability of niacin, lysine, and tryptophan, as well as the calcium content in the grain. It improves flavor, color, and shelf life and limits microbial activity. Additionally, it enhances the variety of food products that can be prepared from maize. For example, in Mexico, more than 300 products are prepared from nixtamalized maize [85, 92, 93]. In Mexico and Central America, maize is consumed mainly in the form of tortillas and related nixtamalized maize-based food products [94]. Apart from nixtamalization, maize is also processed into maize meal, grits, starch, and flour [89]. These are used to prepare other foods, including arepas, cachapas, puddings, porridge, coo coo, broas, baby food, and cereals.

4.3 Aflatoxins in maize and maize products in Latin America and the Caribbean

Maize is one of the most susceptible crops to aflatoxins. The presence of aflatoxins is among the most significant factors affecting local production and international export of maize. The levels of aflatoxigenic fungi and aflatoxin will vary among the countries in the region and intra-country, depending on prevailing environmental, social, and physical conditions during production and processing. In Guatemala, where there is a relatively large production and consumption of maize, the levels of aflatoxins are 10–50 times higher than global averages. This is likely to increase with warming temperatures [95]. An early study in Guatemala showed that the incidence of aflatoxins in maize collected from various locations was 12% (n = 118), with a maximum value of 240 μg/kg. The highest incidence was in the hot, dry zone of the country [96]. Maize cultivated on the Pacific Coast of Guatemala had a similar % contamination incidence of 16% (n = 42) that increased to 24% after two months of storage [97]. Focusing on the highlands of Guatemala, *Aspergillus flavus* was surprisingly present on maize at all farms included in the study, regardless

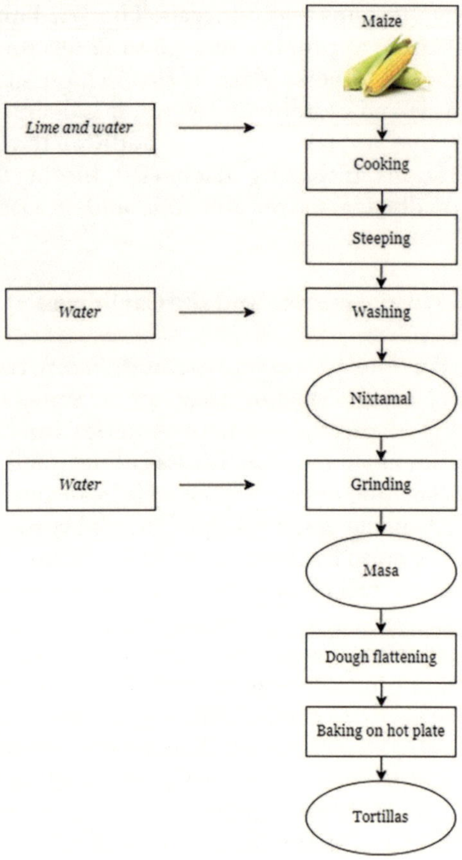

Figure 1.
Scheme of typical steps and intermediate products in traditional maize nixtamalization and tortilla preparation. Source: [91].

of the altitude. Researchers expected that lower incidence levels would be found at higher altitudes where the low temperature could limit the growth and proliferation of the fungus [98]. In another study, aflatoxins were present in maize ranging from 1 to 85 μg/kg with no difference between whether they were purchased or locally produced. It was noted that based on the Provisional Maximum Tolerable Daily Intake (PMTDI) for aflatoxin, consumers' exposure in this area was 280 times the recommended maximum for men and 150 times for women, indicating a significant risk to consumers' health [99]. Similarly, there are concerns about the population's health in Western Honduras since, based on the PMTDI for aflatoxins, exposure was 57 times higher for men and 45 times higher for women [100]. Although a study on freshly harvested maize showed a low aflatoxin incidence of 4.2% (n =24), with the contaminated samples containing aflatoxin concentrations of 6.7 μg/kg and 131.3 μg/kg [101]

In other countries of Latin America and the Caribbean, aflatoxin contamination in maize has been reported at varying levels, ranging from low to very high concentrations. For example, in Columbia, a study on maize and maize products observed concentrations ranging from 2 – 103.3 μg/kg of aflatoxin but a higher incidence of contamination at 12.8% [102]. The high total aflatoxin content of maize found in five different communities of the Columbian Amazon inhabited by three types of Indigenous populations is of even greater significance since there is an increased risk of HCC in this population [80]. In Costa Rica, regional differences were observed in *Aspergillus flavus* and aflatoxin concentration. The high incidence observed in the Brunca region was suggested to result from its relatively higher rainfall and the removal of the maize husks immediately after harvest. The concentration of aflatoxins also increased from harvest through storage and final sale in all the regions [103]. A longitudinal study in that county from 2003 to 2015 investigated the presence of aflatoxins in food and feed, and the results showed 10.8% (n = 5493) incidence in food. Of the 453 white maize samples, 12.4% exceeded Costa Rica's MRL of 20 μg/kg [104]. In Tamaulipas, Mexico, a survey of harvested maize in 1989 detected aflatoxin levels greater than 100 μg/kg, which prompted efforts by the Mexican Government to address the problem [90]. A later study in Tamaulipas utilizing the harvest of 2011 and 2012 and subsequent storage showed that the incidence of *Aspergillus sp*. was approximately 33% (n = 234), and for aflatoxins, less than 2% of the sample exceeded the permissible limit. While this may reflect good management practices as it relates to storage, the presence of *Aspergillus,* and specifically the detection of aflR, aflD, and aflQ genes in those samples, still indicates a risk for potential contamination along the food chain [105]. In a relatively recent study in northwestern Mexico, there were non-detectable levels of AFB_1 in maize from the field and an incidence of 11.1% in market samples, possibly a reflection of the deficiencies in handling [106]. In Haiti, babies are potentially exposed to unhealthy levels of aflatoxin in the maize flour used to prepare food; the mean from the Iron and Relais markets were 5.2 and 32.1 μg/kg, respectively [107].

In Brazil, studies have reported varying results regarding the incidence and concentration of aflatoxin contamination in maize and maize-based products. In one study, aflatoxin incidence in maize was 12.3%, with concentrations ranging from 10 to 900 μg/kg [108]. Similar results were reported in freshly harvested maize in four regions of Brazil (Várzea Grande, Santa Maria, Oliveira dos Campinhos, and Nova Odessa), where the incidence ranged from 2 to 18%, and the highest concentration was 1393 μg/kg [109]. A higher incidence of total aflatoxins (70.8%, n = 24) but with lower concentrations ranging from 0.5 μg/kg to 41.8 μg/kg was detected in another study [110]. However, in the processed maize, no detectable level of aflatoxin was found in maize meal and maize flour traded in São Paulo, Brazil [111]. Using thin-layer chromatography (TLC) and enzyme-linked immunosorbent assay (ELISA), low levels of total aflatoxins were detected at 0.62 μg/kg and 0.78 μg/kg, respectively [112]. These low levels of aflatoxins are perhaps the result of strict implementation of Good Manufacturing Practices (GMPs) [113]. On the other hand, in Rwanda, samples showed a 40% (n = 15) incidence of aflatoxin with a maximum concentration of 15.6 μg/kg [76].

Maize is mechanically harvested when cultivated on a large scale or by hand if planted on small farms. Freshly harvested maize has a high moisture content, so drying must be done using sun drying, solar drying, or mechanical dryers. This reduces the moisture content to prevent microbial growth, including aflatoxigenic fungi and subsequent production of aflatoxins [114]. Drying should be done appropriately and in hygienic conditions to prevent cross-contamination. Sorting is required to remove all debris, damaged kernels, and "fines" that might be a source of inoculum for microbial infection. Storing should be monitored and managed in such a way as to prevent contamination by insects, rodents, and humans [94]. An alternative to the traditional polythene and jute bags for storage is the Purdue Improved Crop Storage (PICS) system, which has been shown to reduce levels of AFB_1 contamination [115]. The PICS is a triple-layer plastic bag that allows dry crops to be stored for an extended period, eliminating the need for insecticides and leading to an overall clean commodity [116]. Other types of hermetically sealed bags, hermetic plastic bags (sBag), and hermetic plastic silo (Bioxilo) were also proven to be better at decreasing insect infestation, reducing fungal growth and subsequent aflatoxin formation than traditional polypropylene sacks [117]. Despite the hermetic seal, frequent opening of containers should be discouraged since fungal growth and subsequent aflatoxin contamination may occur [118]. However, the high quality of PICS facilitates repeated opening and reuse of the bags [119].

During storage, maize can be chemically treated to control aflatoxin contamination. Naturally contaminated maize treated with sodium bisulfite (0.5%), NaOH (0.5%), or ammonia, then stored for 24 hours at ambient temperatures reduced AFB_1 and AFB_2. There was a direct relationship between the $NaHSO_3$ concentrations that vary from 0.5 to 2% and total aflatoxin degradation. However, for highly contaminated maize, increased concentration and increased treatment time were required for effective aflatoxin destruction. The sodium bisulfite converts the aflatoxin into water-soluble forms, resulting in its degradation [120, 121].

Maize processing in its various forms can reduce the levels of aflatoxins. Process conditions that include the application of heat (boiling, baking, and frying) and/or pH changes can limit the presence of aflatoxins in foods. Naturally contaminated maize, when made into grits by grinding the raw maize and then boiling, showed a reduction in aflatoxin contamination, between 21% and 28%, while frying of the grits reduced aflatoxin by 34–61%. When the same naturally contaminated maize was ground and then used for baking muffins, aflatoxin reduction was reported to be between 13% and 17% [122]. In Ethiopia, when the maize was first dried and then soaked in 300 ml of cold water before boiling, a higher reduction of aflatoxin levels was observed, ranging from 88.6 to 89.9% [123].

Among the factors influencing the degree to which fermentation reduces mycotoxins in maize are the type of bacteria, substrate type, and incubation time. Lactic acid bacteria formed during natural fermentation of both hulled and dehulled maize reduced aflatoxins by physical absorption, binding to the toxins. However, *Lactobacillus fermentum* or a combination of *Lactobacillus fermentum* and *Lactobacillus plantarum* increased AFB1 and AFB2, possibly because of the formation and reformation of the lactone ring [124].

Application of various pH levels to maize during processing can substantially reduce aflatoxins. Apart from enhanced maize nutrition, the alkalinity in nixtamalization and its multiple modifications may reduce aflatoxin in maize. Alkalinity opens the lactone ring of aflatoxin B_1, essential to its toxicity, to form a substitute o-coumaric acid. Naturally contaminated maize and maize containing radioactively labeled aflatoxin were both subjected to the traditional nixtamalization process, which involves washing the maize to remove debris, followed by covering the maize with water containing 10 g of lime. The mixture was boiled for 50 minutes or until turbid, then steeped for 17 hours. After the resting period, the water was removed, and the maize was ground to form masa used to produce tortillas. Results showed a 100% aflatoxin reduction in less contaminated aflatoxin-contaminated maize and a 97% reduction in samples with relatively higher contamination. A reduction of 84% was observed in the samples containing radioactively labeled aflatoxin [125]. Washing to partially remove the maize pericarp, followed by nixtamalization, facilitated the reduction of aflatoxin B_1 by 94% [126]. Efforts to improve the nixtamalization process by making it more ecologically friendly by using less lime, higher boiling temperature, and steeping for less time demonstrated that the traditional process achieved a higher level of reduction [127]. Recommendations for improving the efficacy of nixtamalization and reducing AFB_1 include a ratio of 1 part calcium hydroxide to 300 parts water, cooking for more than 40 minutes, no less than 6 hours steeping, followed by washing the nixtamal. In their survey, the researchers found that most households wash the nixtamal thrice [128]. At pH 10.2, there was a total reduction (100%) of aflatoxin in spiked masa dough, while for the unspiked dough, it was 97.7% [129]. In making maize products, there is a progressive decline in aflatoxin concentration from the raw material through production to nixtamal, masa, tortilla, tortilla chips, and maize chips. Cooking, steeping, baking, frying, and other necessary steps contribute to aflatoxin reduction in maize-based products. The different processes and processing parameters (time and temperature) applied in making tortillas, tortilla chips, and maize chips resulted in the elimination of 51.7%, 84.5%, and 78.8% of aflatoxin, respectively, compared to the initial maize contamination [130]. A similar trend in reduction was observed in four communities in Honduras, where there was a progressive decline in aflatoxins throughout the tortilla-making process. From the maize kernels to masa, the reduction ranged from 72.8 to 76.3%, and from masa to tortilla, aflatoxin reductions from 46.8 to 51.4% were observed. The overall reduction from kernels to tortillas was 81.5–83.3% [131]. Tortilla gathered from five departments in Guatemala also indicated a reduction of 58.8% of aflatoxin contamination when compared to maize [132]. Nixtamalization, as a strategy to reduce aflatoxins and improve the functionality of maize, is also being applied in other parts of the world, such as Rwanda [133]. In Kenya, it was determined that primary school children are exposed to potentially dangerous levels of aflatoxins in meals through the school feeding program. Nixtamalization was demonstrated to be an effective strategy to reduce aflatoxin exposure [134].

Nixtamalization, in concert with other strategies, is also effective at minimizing aflatoxins in foods. A modified tortilla-making process in which spiked maize mixed with water and lime was microwaved before steeping resulted in a reduction of up to 84% of aflatoxins and, even more significant, extract acidification where the masa and tortilla extracts from the aflatoxin assay were adjusted to pH 3 to simulate stomach acidity resulted in almost eliminating aflatoxins [135]. Infrared heating applied to maize contaminated with 175 μg/kg and 370 μg/kg reduced aflatoxin levels by 71% and 73%, respectively. When the maize was processed into tortilla, there was a further reduction of 15% and 25%, respectively [136].

Baking the nixtamalized maize flour contributes to reducing aflatoxins. While calcium hydroxide was the most effective alkali solution when compared to ashes, tequesquite—a mineral salt, and calcium chloride in preparing maize bread from nixtamalized maize, it was the baking process at 200°C for 20 minutes that caused the highest percentage of reduction [137].

Extrusion cooking applies mechanical and shear forces to food material through a heated barrel for a specific amount of time, with the final product exiting through a die to achieve the required form [138]. While extrusion was not intended to serve as a decontamination method, the features of the process enable the destruction of aflatoxin. Extrusion of instant maize porridge and chapatti showed that there is a direct relationship between temperature and AFB_1 reduction but an indirect relationship between moisture content and AFB_1 reduction and extruder screw speed and AFB1 reduction. The maximum aflatoxin reduction was obtained at 24% moisture, 171°C temperature, and a screw speed of 369 rpm [139]. Extrusion of maize meal using an extruder screw with a compression ratio of 3:1, a length-to-diameter ratio of 20:1, and speeds of 160 and 210 rpm achieved a significant reduction of AFB_1 (82.1–91.1%); AFB_2 (79.9–88.8%); AFG_1 (70.8–78.3%); and AFG_2 (84.1–95.2%) [140]. Extrusion of nixtamalized maize with or without chemicals can reduce aflatoxin in the final product. Extrusion of nixtamalized ground maize with various concentrations of lime showed a direct relationship between the reduction of aflatoxin and lime concentrations. Among the concentrations of lime applied, the highest reduction (85%) was observed, with 0.5% lime added to the extrusion process. When hydrogen peroxide was added to the extrusion process, 0.3% lime and 0.75% hydrogen peroxide (H_2O_2) resulted in undetectable aflatoxin B1 [126].

Despite maize processing potentially reducing aflatoxin contamination of maize-based products, evidence indicates that the high consumption of these foods may still lead to exposure that presents a health risk. In Mexico, total aflatoxins were detected at an incidence of 17% (n = 396) ranging from 3 to 385 μg/kg in nixtamalized tortillas. AFB_1 was found in 64.6% of tortillas analyzed at levels ranging from 3.0 to 140.3 μg/kg. In Guatemala, research has shown a direct relationship between AFB_1-lysine adduct and tortilla consumption among adults, which is concerning. Further, in Mexico, the estimated cancer risk is greater than one in a million upon lifetime exposure, indicating a potentially harmful exposure. AFB_1 exposure via nixtamalized products might account for between 0.2% and 10.5% of the HCC cases. Hence, efforts should be made to reduce contamination of maize-based products with aflatoxin by utilizing only high-quality and safe maize during processing. Specifically associated with nixtamalization, the reuse of water should be avoided [132, 141–144].

5. Rice as a staple food in Latin America and the Caribbean

Spanish colonists first introduced Rice (*Oryza sativa*) in Latin America and the Caribbean in the sixteenth century. Rice has since become a widely cultivated crop, and about twenty-six countries in Latin America and the Caribbean commercially cultivate rice. In this region, rice is grown in a range of conditions, from the semi-tropical and temperate regions of Brazil, Uruguay, and Argentina to the irrigated upland of Central America and Mexico. Rice has become increasingly important in Latin America and the Caribbean. It provides more calories to the human diet than wheat, maize, cassava, and potatoes. The production of rice has increased exponentially even without direct expansion in the cultivation area. This is largely the result of high-yielding varieties, but demand still exceeds supply, so Latin America and the Caribbean continue to be a net importer of rice [145–147]. In the year 2022, Brazil had the highest production of rice in Latin America and the Caribbean region with over 10 million tonnes, followed by Peru with more than 3 million tonnes, then Columbia produced over 2 million tonnes [45], as displayed in **Table 1**.

5.1 Nutritional composition of rice

Rice is an excellent carbohydrate source, accounting for about 80% of its composition. The carbohydrates in rice are stored primarily as starch. Additionally, rice consists of about 7–8% protein, 3% lipids, and 3% fiber, and is also a good source of vitamins B and minerals [148]. However, the nutritional composition of rice may vary based on the variety of rice and the growing conditions. Further, the processing techniques to produce white rice (dehulled, bran, and germ removed), brown rice (dehulled, bran, and germ layers remained), and parboiled rice (partially boiled in the husk before milling) also have a significant effect on the nutrient composition of rice [149]. Brown rice retains the bran and germ layers, so it is superior to white rice in protein, lipids, and other associated micronutrients.

Rice has a high proportion of lysine and high protein digestibility [148]. Other amino acids include histidine, isoleucine, leucine, phenylalanine, and tryptophan. The vitamins present are mainly thiamine, riboflavin, niacin, and tocopherol. The essential B vitamins found in rice are primarily located in the germ and bran layer and are removed during milling. The process used to produce white rice removes approximately 80% of the thiamine and other essential nutrients found in the bran [150]. Rice also contains essential minerals, including phosphorus, potassium, magnesium, calcium, iron, and zinc [151]. The application of genetic engineering has enabled its fortification with nutrients such as β-carotene and zinc [148].

The health benefits of rice include its anti-inflammatory and anti-cancer properties. Rice also controls blood cholesterol and reduces the risk of heart disease. However, rice consumption may also present some risks. For example, since rice is grown in flooded conditions, there is the possibility of arsenic uptake, which is a metal dangerous to human health, with an increased risk for cancer and other harmful effects [152]. High consumption of rice raises the glycemic index and consequently increases the chance of developing diabetes [153].

5.2 Aflatoxins in rice in Latin America and the Caribbean

There have been fewer studies on aflatoxins in rice in Latin America and the Caribbean compared to maize. In most countries, paddy rice is cultivated under flooded conditions and harvested when dry. At harvest, the paddy moisture content is usually high. Drying should reduce the moisture content initially at 22–25% moisture to about 14% before milling [154].

The harvested paddy is cleaned and then mechanically processed by milling into various fractions, with the first dehulling forming brown rice, which is further milled to prepare white rice and bran. In Brazil, an investigation determined the presence of aflatoxigenic fungi and aflatoxins in the soil used for rice production and in milled fractions of rice available at markets when the rice was grown in wetland farms in Rio Grande do Sul and dryland farms in Maranhão. The soil was contaminated with *Aspergillus* section *Flavi,* occurring at a higher incidence in the dryland than in the wetland. For the rice, mold infection was directly related to the water activity of the grain. Aflatoxigenic fungal infection in rice samples decreased during the drying and processing stages in both areas as the paddy was de-husked, polished, and/or parboiled. For the market collection, some red and black rice samples showed higher mold infection rates than others (polished, brown, and parboiled). The rice products, which included paddy rice, rice husks, husked rice, polished rice, brown, red, parboiled rice, rice flour, and red and flake rice, had no detectable levels of aflatoxin. Bran, however, had low levels of aflatoxin [155]. Bran was also found to have the highest concentration of total aflatoxins by other researchers [156], but in this latter study, all fractions had detectable levels of aflatoxins. In a northwestern region of Mexico, an investigation of AFB_1 contamination in paddy rice revealed an incidence of 21.2% (n = 43), with levels ranging from 2.27 to 47.07 μg/kg. At the same time, none was detected in polished rice sold in the market [106]. In Guyana, a study on paddy at the farm level, paddy at the mill, and subsequent fractions (steamed paddy, white rice, parboiled rice, and cargo/brown rice) found that the overall aflatoxin incidence was 8.2% (n = 182). However, for samples of white and parboiled rice collected from markets, the incidence was 5.1% (n = 117). Regarding the fractions, the highest incidence was associated with parboiled rice at 26.3% (n = 19) and steamed paddy at 25% (n = 8). Since water is used in both processes, water activity and moisture likely influenced fungal growth [75]. Parboiled rice is prepared by steeping the rice overnight in water. Depending on steeping time, there is migration of aflatoxins into the rice kernels [157–159]. Similarly, in Pakistan, an investigation of aflatoxin contamination in rice revealed high levels of aflatoxin in paddy rice and much lower levels in white rice produced after several fractions [160]. Storage and handling conditions before milling and during milling can impact aflatoxin levels. During milling, the sequential stages facilitate the refining and removal of aflatoxins.

In Brazil, research further evaluated the risk of ingesting foods with aflatoxin. For rice, the incidence was reported as 37.6% (n = 202). The margin of exposure was 25.8–25.0, and the cancer risk was 0.0731–0.0753 per year per 10 individuals. This cancer risk is much higher than the one estimated for Europe but lower than for Africa [113]. These concerns are supported by other studies in Brazil, where the incidence of contamination by total aflatoxins in rice was 45.1% (n = 166), with 11.4% above the maximum tolerable limit of 5 µg/kg [161]. Other reports showed that the incidence of contamination with total aflatoxin in rice was 58.7% (n = 230), with levels in the range of 0.11–207.04 µg/kg and a mean contamination value of 13.13 µg/kg. AFB_1 was the most common aflatoxin. Rice husk and rice bran had a higher incidence of contamination than other rice products [28]. Organically-produced rice fractions in Brazil—parboiled, polished, and whole grain—might be an alternative to traditional farming methods since it was observed that all fractions of organically-produced rice had aflatoxin levels below the maximum tolerable limit of 5 µg/kg. Despite this, there are still concerns about consumers' health given Brazil's high rice consumption and average probable daily intake of aflatoxins [162].

Rice must be cooked before consumption and preparation methods can impact aflatoxin contamination. As far as possible, the methods should be practicable and preserve the organoleptic quality of the rice. In Latin America and the Caribbean, consumers cook rice by boiling it in excess water, with the remaining water being drained when the rice is cooked, or by boiling with just enough water so that all is absorbed during the cooking process. The latter can be done using a rice cooker. Studies comparing the effect of draining the excess water from cooked rice with that of a rice cooker showed that aflatoxin reduction occurred in both methods. When excess water is removed upon cooking, aflatoxins may have drained with the cooking water, and contamination was decreased by 17.5%. However, with the cooker, aflatoxin may have been carried out by the evaporating steam during cooking, achieving reductions as high as 24.8% [163]. Boiling white and brown rice spiked with AFB_1, AFB_2, AFG_1, and AFG_2 at 100°C for 12 mins resulted in losses of 30%, 38%, 25%, and 29% in white rice for the respective aflatoxins and 49%, 56%, 36%, and 40% in brown rice. Pressure cooking of rice is less common; however, the reduction of total aflatoxin contamination achieved with this method is much higher at 78–88%. The high pressure allows the processing at increased temperatures, leading to greater degradation of aflatoxins. At high temperatures, the lactone ring of the coumarin moiety in the aflatoxin molecule is easily hydrolyzed by water, causing its degradation [164, 165]. High aflatoxin reductions ranging from 81 to 91% were also observed when brown, parboiled, and polished rice were hydrothermally treated and then cooked either in a microwave or a hot plate [166].

6. Conclusion

Aflatoxins are present in cassava, maize, and rice, as well as their products, throughout their production and processing chains in Latin America and the Caribbean. Although the levels may be low in some cases, the high consumption of these foods increases the risk to human health with the potential for developing chronic or acute conditions. This can significantly impact food security in local communities and nationally. Hence, efforts should be focused on developing cost-effective and sustainable strategies to limit the contamination of foods throughout the production and marketing chain. In addition, governments should implement policies to safeguard consumers while providing training and raising awareness among farmers and processors about the risks associated with fungal contamination and mycotoxins. Only an integrated approach where farmers, the food industry, and regulators collaborate will improve food safety and security in these areas of the world while safeguarding consumers' health.

Author details

Donna M. Morrison[1]*, Ram K. Shrestha[2] and Andréia Bianchini[2]

1 Faculty of Agriculture and Forestry, University of Guyana, Turkeyen, Greater Georgetown, Guyana

2 Department of Food Science and Technology, University of Nebraska-Lincoln, Lincoln, NE, USA

*Address all correspondence to: donna.morrison@uog.edu.gy

References

[1] Quam J, Campbell S. The Western World: Daily Readings in Geography. Illinois, US: College DuPage Digital Press; 2020

[2] Kovalskys I, Fisberg M, Gómez G, Pareja R, García MC, Sanabria LY, et al. Energy intake and food sources of eight Latin American countries: Results from the Latin American study of nutrition and health (ELANS). Public Health Nutrition. 2018;**21**(14):2535-2547

[3] Tanumihardjo SA, McCulley L, Roh R, Lopez-Ridaura S, Palacios-Rojas N, Gunaratna NS. Maize agro-food systems to ensure food and nutrition security in reference to the sustainable development goals. Global Food Security. 2020;**25**:100327

[4] Inter-American Development Bank. Food Security in Latin America and the Caribbean [Internet]. Washington, DC: Inter-American Development Bank; 2024. Available from: Food Security in Latin America and the Caribbean

[5] FAO, IFAD, UNICEF, WFP, WHO. The State of Food Security and Nutrition in the World 2024 – Financing to End Hunger, Food Insecurity and Malnutrition in all its Forms [Internet]. Rome, Italy; 2024. Available from: https://openknowledge.fao.org/handle/20.500.14283/cd1254en

[6] Robertson K, Ellsworth B. Can the Caribbean farm its way out of reliance on food imports? Americas Quarterly [Internet]. 2024. Available from: https://www.americasquarterly.org/article/can-the-caribbean-farm-its-way-out-of-reliance-on-food-imports/

[7] FAO. The State of Food Insecurity in the World 2001. [Internet]. Rome, Italy; 2002. Available from: https://www.fao.org/4/y1500e/y1500e00.htm

[8] WHO. Food safety [Internet]. 2025. Available from: https://www.who.int/health-topics/food-safety

[9] Bennett JW, Klich M. Mycotoxins. Clinical Microbiology Reviews. 2003;**16**(3):497-516

[10] Gruber-Dorninger C, Jenkins T, Schatzmayr G. Global mycotoxin occurrence in feed: A Ten-year survey. Toxins. 2019;**11**(7):375

[11] International Agency for Research on Cancer Working Group. IARC monographs 100F [Internet]. 2002. Available from: http://www.iarc.fr/

[12] Kabak B. The fate of mycotoxins during thermal food processing. Journal of the Science of Food and Agriculture. 2009;**89**(4):549-554

[13] Cotty PJ, Jaime-Garcia R. Influences of climate on aflatoxin producing fungi and aflatoxin contamination. International Journal of Food Microbiology. 2007;**119**(1-2):109-115

[14] Tesfamariam K, De Boevre M, Kolsteren P, Belachew T, Mesfin A, De Saeger S, et al. Dietary mycotoxins exposure and child growth, immune system, morbidity, and mortality: A systematic literature review. Critical Reviews in Food Science and Nutrition. 2020;**60**(19):3321-3341

[15] Kensler TW, Roebuck BD, Wogan GN, Groopman JD. Aflatoxin: A 50-year odyssey of mechanistic and translational. Toxicological Sciences. 2011;**120**(S1):S28-S48

[16] Kumar A, Pathak H, Bhadauria S, Sudan J. Aflatoxin contamination in food crops: Causes, detection, and management: A review. Food Production, Processing and Nutrition. 2021;**3**:1-9

[17] Solís-Martínez O, Monge A, Groopman JD, McGlynn KA, Romero M, Palacios-Rojas N, et al. Maize consumption and circulating aflatoxin levels in Mexican middle- and older-aged adults: A cross-sectional analysis. The American Journal of Clinical Nutrition. 2025;**121**(2):454-462

[18] Marin S, Ramos AJ, Cano-Sancho G, Sanchis V. Mycotoxins: Occurrence, toxicology, and exposure assessment. Food and Chemical Toxicology. 2013;**60**:218-237

[19] Williams JH, Aggarwal D, Phillips TD, Jolly PE, Stiles JK, Jolly CM. Human aflatoxicosis in developing countries: A review of toxicology, exposure, potential health consequences, and interventions. American Journal of Clinical Nutrition. 2004;**80**:1106-1122

[20] Shephard GS. Determination of mycotoxins in human foods. Chemical Society Reviews. 2008;**37**:2468-2477

[21] Goss PE, Lee BL, Badovinac-Crnjevic T, Strasser-Weippl K, Chavarri-Guerra Y, St Louis J, et al. Planning cancer control in Latin America. Lancet Oncology. 2013;**14**:391-436

[22] Torres O, Matute J, Gelineau-van Waes J, Maddox JR, Gregory SG, Ashley-Koch AE, et al. Human health implications from co-exposure to aflatoxins and fumonisins in maize-based foods in Latin America: Guatemala as a case study. WMJ. 2015;**8**:143-160

[23] Smith JW, Kroker-Lobos MF, Lazo M, Rivera-Andrade A, Egner PA, Wedemeyer H, et al. Aflatoxin and viral hepatitis exposures in Guatemala: Molecular biomarkers reveal a unique profile of risk factors in a region of high liver cancer incidence. PLoS One. 2017;**12**(12):e0189255

[24] Coppa CFSC, Cirelli AC, Gonçalves BL, Barnabé EMB, Mousavi Khaneghah A, Corassin CH, et al. Dietary exposure assessment and risk characterization of mycotoxins in lactating women: Case study of São Paulo state, Brazil. Food Research International. 2020;**134**:109272

[25] Brown LR. Aflatoxins in Food and Feed Impacts, Risks, and Management Strategies [Internet]. The US Government's Hunger Global Hunger and Food Security Initiative; 2018. (Gender, Climate Change, and Nutrition Integration Initiative (GCAN)). Report No.: 9. Available from: https://gcan.ifpri.info/files/2018/07/GCAN-Aflatoxins_Note-9_web.pdf

[26] Liu Y, Wu F. Global burden of aflatoxin-induced hepatocellular carcinoma: A risk assessment. Environmental Health Perspectives. 2010;**118**:818-824

[27] Wu F, Narrod C, Tiongco M, Liu Y. The Health Economics of Aflatoxin: Global Burden of Disease. Washington, DC: IFPRI; 2011

[28] Almeida MI, Almeida NG, Carvalho KL, Gonçalves GAA, Silva CN, Santos EA, et al. Co-occurrence of aflatoxins B1, B2, G1 and G2, ochratoxin a, zearalenone, deoxynivalenol, and citreoviridin in rice in Brazil. Food Additives and Contaminants - Part A Chemistry, Analysis, Control, Exposure and Risk Assessment. 2012;**29**:694-703

[29] Voth-Gaeddert LE, Torres O, Maldonado J, Krajmalnik-Brown R, Rittmann BE, Oerther DB. Aflatoxin

exposure, child stunting, and dysbiosis in the intestinal microbiome among children in Guatemala. Environmental Engineering Science. 2019;**36**:958-968

[30] Jolly PE, Mazariegos M, Contreras H, Balas N, Junkins A, Aina IO, et al. Aflatoxin exposure among mothers and their infants from the Western highlands of Guatemala. Maternal and Child Health Journal. 2021;**25**:1316-1325

[31] Kelly JD, Eaton DL, Guengerich FP, Coulombe RA. Aflatoxin B1 activation in human lung. Toxicology and Applied Pharmacology. 1997;**144**:88-95

[32] Yang XJ, Lu HY, Li ZY, Bian Q, Qiu LL, Li Z, et al. Cytochrome P450 2A13 mediates aflatoxin B1-induced cytotoxicity and apoptosis in human bronchial epithelial cells. Toxicology. 2012;**300**:138-148

[33] Food and Agriculture Organization. Worldwide regulations for mycotoxins in food and feed [internet]. FAO. Food and Nutrition. 2004. Report No.: 81. Available from: https://www.fao.org/4/y5499e/y5499e00.htm

[34] Scussel VM. Aflatoxin and food safety: Recent south American perspectives. Journal of Toxicology: Toxin Reviews. 2004;**23**:179-216

[35] Wu F, Stacy SL, Kensler TW. Global assessment of aflatoxins in maize and peanuts: Are regulatory standards adequately protective? Toxicological Letters. 2013;**135**:251-259

[36] Cardwell KF, Desjardins A, Henry SH, Munkvold G, Robens J. Mycotoxins: The Cost of Achieving Food Security and Food Quality [Internet]. 2001. DOI: 10.1094/APSnetFeature-2001-0901

[37] International Agency for Research on Cancer. Improving public health through mycotoxin control. Lyon, France: International Agency for Research on Cancer (IARC Scientific Publications Series, No. 158). In: IARC Scientific Publications Series [Internet]. 2012:119-129. Available from: https://linkinghub.elsevier.com/retrieve/pii/S0278691512007302

[38] Jackson J, Chiwona-Karltun L, Gordon A. Food safety and quality considerations for cassava, a major staple containing a natural toxicant. In: Food Safety and Quality Systems in Developing Countries [Internet]. Elsevier; 2020. pp. 343-366. Available from: https://linkinghub.elsevier.com/retrieve/pii/B9780128142721000085

[39] FAO, Clayuca Corporation, IICA. Cassava in the Caribbean Region [Internet]. FAO, Clayuca Corporation, IICA; 2016. Available from: https://repositorio.iica.int/bitstream/handle/

[40] Alves AAC. Cassava botany and physiology. In: Hillocks RJ, Thresh JM, editors. Cassava: Biology, Production and Utilization [Internet]. 1st ed. UK: CABI Publishing; 2001. pp. 67-89. DOI: 10.1079/9780851995243.0067

[41] Parmar A, Sturm B, Hensel O. Crops that feed the world: Production and improvement of cassava for food, feed, and industrial uses. Food Security. 2017;**9**:907-927

[42] Ferraro V, Piccirillo C, Tomlins K, Pintado ME. Cassava (*Manihot esculenta* Crantz) and yam (*Dioscorea* spp.) crops and their derived foodstuffs: Safety, security and nutritional value. Critical Reviews in Food Science and Nutrition. 2016;**56**:2714-2727

[43] Henry G, Hershey C. Cassava in South America and the Caribbean. In: Hillocks RJ, Thresh JM, editors. Cassava: Biology, Production and

Utilization [Internet]. 1st ed. UK: CABI Publishing; 2001. pp. 17-40. DOI: 10.1079/9780851995243.0017

[44] Vilpoux OF, De Oliveira GD, Pascoli CM. Cassava cultivation in Latin America. In: Formerly International Center for Tropical Agriculture (CIAT), Colombia, Hershey C, editors. Achieving Sustinable Cultivation of Cassava [Internet]. Burleigh Dodds Science Publishing; 2017. pp. 149-174. Available from: https://shop.bdspublishing.com/store/bds/detail/product/3-190-9781838790561

[45] FAO. Crop Production Statistics. 2023

[46] Montagnac JA, Davis CR, Tanumihardjo SA. Nutritional value of cassava for use as a staple food and recent advances for improvement. Comprehensive Reviews in Food Science and Food Safety. 2009;**8**:181-194

[47] Scaria SS, Balasubramanian B, Meyyazhagan A, Gangwar J, Jaison JP, Kurian JT, et al. Cassava (*Manihot esculenta* Crantz)—A potential source of phytochemicals, food, and nutrition—An updated review. eFood. 2024;**5**:e127

[48] Wang Z, Mhaske P, Farahnaky A, Kasapis S, Majzoobi M. Cassava starch: Chemical modification and its impact on functional properties and digestibility, a review. Food Hydrocolloids. 2022;**129**:107542

[49] Astley S, Finglas P. Nutrition and health. In: Reference Module in Food Science [Internet]. Elsevier; 2016. p. B9780081005965034259. Available from: https://linkinghub.elsevier.com/retrieve/pii/B9780081005965034259

[50] Gleadow RM, Møller BL. Cyanogenic glycosides: Synthesis, physiology, and phenotypic plasticity. Annual Review of Plant Biology. 2014;**65**:155-185

[51] Teles FFF. Chronic poisoning by hydrogen cyanide in cassava and its prevention in Africa and Latin America. Food and Nutrition Bulletin. 2002;**23**:407-412

[52] Alitubeera PH, Eyu P, Kwesiga B, Ario AR, Zhu BP. Outbreak of cyanide poisoning caused by consumption of cassava flour—Kasese District, Uganda, September 2017. MMWR. Morbidity and Mortality Weekly Report. 2019;**68**:308-311

[53] Egbune EO, Ezedom T, Orororo OC, Egbune OU, Avwioroko OJ, Aganbi E, et al. Solid-state fermentation of cassava (*Manihot esculenta* Crantz): A review. World Journal of Microbiology and Biotechnology. 2023;**39**:259

[54] Qi M, Song J, Jiang L, Li L, Xu M, Li Y, et al. Understanding the degradation mechanisms of cyanide and starch in cassava flour during extrusion processing. Innovative Food Science and Emerging Technologies. 2024;**91**:103548

[55] Quinn AA, Myrans H, Gleadow RM. Cyanide content of cassava food products available in Australia. Food. 2022;**11**:1384

[56] Thaweewong P, Anuntagool J. Change in free cyanide content of bitter cassava during incubation and drying and physical properties of dry-milled cassava flour. Food and Bioproducts Processing. 2023;**138**:139-149

[57] Ono LT, Taniwaki MH. Fungi and mycotoxins in cassava (*Manihot esculenta* Crantz) and its products. Brazilian Journal of Food Technology. 2021;**24**:e2020240

[58] Sharma K, Kaur R, Kumar S, Saini RK, Sharma S, Pawde SV, et al. Saponins: A concise review on food-related aspects, applications and health

implications. Food Chemistry Advances. 2023;**2**:100191

[59] Wobeto C, Corrêa AD, de Abreu CMP, dos Santos CD, Pereira HV. Antinutrients in the cassava (*Manihot esculenta* Crantz) leaf powder at three ages of the plant. Food Science and Technology (Campinas). 2007;**27**:108-112

[60] Price RK, Welch RW. Cereal grains. In: Encyclopedia of Human Nutrition. Cambridge: Academic Press; 2013. pp. 307-316

[61] Mariam LW, Woldeyes F. Review on effect of processing on cassava anti-nutritional factors and impacts on health. IJFR [Internet]. 2020;**1**(1). Available from: https://www.opastonline.com/wp-content/uploads/2020/11/review-on-effect-of-processing-on-cassava-anti-nutritional-factors-and-impacts-on-health-ijfr-20.pdf

[62] Brimer L. Cassava production and processing and impact on biological compounds. In: Processing and Impact of Active Components in Food. London: Academic Press; 2015. pp. 81-88

[63] Crenn J. Cassava products of Brazil. IFAD - West and Central Africa Division. 2020:1-13. Available from: cassava-ipci.nri.org

[64] Oliveira LA d. Processing of Sweet and Bitter Cassava. Brasília, DF: Embrapa; 2021

[65] Duford D. Journey by bottle: Discovering the allure of Guyanese Casareep. Gastronomica. 2012;**12**(4):27-30

[66] Ramos CL, Schwan RF. Technological and nutritional aspects of indigenous Latin America fermented foods. Current Opinion in Food Science. 2017;**13**:97-102

[67] Ono LT, Silva JJ, Doná S, Martins LM, Iamanaka BT, Fungaro MHP, et al. Aspergillus section Flavi and aflatoxins in Brazilian cassava (*Manihot esculenta* Crantz) and products. Mycotoxin Research. 2021;**37**:221-228

[68] Adjovi YCS, Bailly S, Gnonlonfin BJG, Tadrist S, Querin A, Sanni A, et al. Analysis of the contrast between natural occurrence of toxigenic aspergilli of the Flavi section and aflatoxin B1 in cassava. Food Microbiology. 2014;**38**:151-159

[69] Mundim SM, Kluczkovski AM, Rodrigues JC, Brito VH, Fernandes OC. Cyanide influence on the growth of mycotoxigenic fungi from cassava flour in vitro. African Journal of Microbiology Research. 2015;**9**:1184-1188

[70] Kaaya AN, Eboku D. Mould and aflatoxin contamination of dried cassava chips with traditional processing and storage practices. Journal of Biological Sciences. 2010;**10**:718-729

[71] Essono G, Ayodele M, Akoa A, Foko J, Filtenborg O, Olembo S. Aflatoxin-producing aspergillus spp. and aflatoxin levels in stored cassava chips as affected by processing practices. Food Control. 2009;**20**:648-654

[72] Oyesigye E, Cervini C, Mahuku G, Medina A. Potential impact of current agricultural practices on mycotoxin occurrence and mycotoxin knowledge along the cassava value chain in Uganda. Journal of Food Protection. 2024;**87**:100340

[73] Alamu EO, Gondwe T, Ayinde O, Akinwale G, Ntawuruhunga P, Awoyale W, et al. Physicochemical, microbial, and aflatoxin analyses of selected high-quality cassava flour (HQCF) from the major markets of Zambia. Cogent Food & Agriculture. 2021;**7**:1914906

[74] Kluczkovski AM, Diogenes L, Barroncas J, Silva A, Torres TV, Lima E, et al. Aflatoxins in tapioca gum marketed in Manaus-AM-Brazil. JFR. 2024;**13**:1

[75] Morrison DM, Ledoux DR, Chester LFB, Samuels CAN. Occurrence of aflatoxins in rice and in cassava (Manihot esculenta) products (meal, bread) produced in Guyana. Mycotoxin Research. 2019;**35**:75-81

[76] Matsiko F, Kanyange C, Ingabire G, Dusingizimana T, Vasanthakaalam H, Kimonyo A. Detection and quantification of aflatoxin in cassava and maize flour sold. International Food Research. 2017;**24**:459-464

[77] Udomkun P, Mutegi C, Wossen T, Atehnkeng J, Nabahungu NL, Njukwe E, et al. Occurrence of aflatoxin in agricultural produce from local markets in Burundi and eastern Democratic Republic of Congo. Food Science & Nutrition. 2018;**6**:2227-2238

[78] Udomkun P, Tirawattanawanich C, Ilukor J, Sridonpai P, Njukwe E, Nimbona P, et al. Promoting the use of locally produced crops in making cereal-legume-based composite flours: An assessment of nutrient, antinutrient, mineral molar ratios, and aflatoxin content. Food Chemistry. 2019;**286**:651-658

[79] Muzanila YC, Brennan JG, King RD. Residual cyanogens, chemical composition and aflatoxins in cassava flour from Tanzanian villages. Food Chemistry. 2000;**70**:45-49

[80] Diaz GJ, Krska R, Sulyok M. Mycotoxins and cyanogenic glycosides in staple foods of three indigenous people of the Colombian Amazon. Food Additives & Contaminants: Part B. 2015:**8**(4):291-297

[81] Gnonlonfin GJB, Adjovi CSY, Katerere DR, Shephard GS, Sanni A, Brimer L. Mycoflora and absence of aflatoxin contamination of commercialized cassava chips in Benin, West Africa. Food Control. 2012;**23**:333-337

[82] Guzzon F, Arandia Rios LW, Caviedes Cepeda GM, Céspedes Polo M, Chavez Cabrera A, Muriel Figueroa J, et al. Conservation and use of Latin American maize diversity: Pillar of nutrition security and cultural heritage of humanity. Agronomy. 2021;**11**:172

[83] Bedoya CA, Dreisigacker S, Hearne S, Franco J, Mir C, Prasanna BM, et al. Genetic diversity and population structure of native maize populations in Latin America and the Caribbean. PLoS One. 2017;**12**(4):e0173488

[84] Mickleburgh HL, Pagán-Jiménez JR. New insights into the consumption of maize and other food plants in the pre-Columbian Caribbean from starch grains trapped in human dental calculus. Journal of Archaeological Science. 2012;**39**(7):2468-2478

[85] Staller JE. Maize in Andean food and culture: Interdisciplinary approaches. In: Staller JE, editor. Andean Foodways [Internet]. Cham: Springer International Publishing; 2021. pp. 283-310. (The Latin American Studies Book Series). DOI: 10.1007/978-3-030-51629-1_11

[86] Wu F, Narrod C, Tiongco M, Liu Y. The health economics of aflatoxin: Global burden of disease. Afla Control. 2011;**4**:1-14

[87] Klein HS, Luna FV. The impact of the rise of modern maize production in Brazil and Argentina. HIST AGRAR [Internet]. 2022. Available from: https://www.historiaagraria.com/FILE/articulos/RHA86-klein-vidal.pdf

[88] Loy DD, Lundy EL. Nutritional properties and feeding value of corn and its coproducts. In: Corn Chemistry and Technology. Third. Cereals and Grains Association. Amsterdam: Elsevier Inc; 2003. pp. 633-659

[89] Rouf, Shah T, Prasad K, Kumar P. Maize—A potential source of human nutrition and health: A review. Cogent Food & Agriculture [Internet]. 2016;**2**(1):1166995

[90] Plasencia J. Aflatoxins in maize: A Mexican perspective. Journal of Toxicology: Toxin Reviews. 2004;**23**:155-177

[91] Schaarschmidt S, Fauhl-Hassek C. Mycotoxins during the processes of nixtamalization and tortilla production. Toxins. 2019;**11**:227

[92] Santiago-Ramos D, Figueroa-Cardenas J, Mariscal-Moreno RM, Escalante-Aburto A, Ponce-García N, Veles-Medina JJ. Physical and chemical changes undergone by pericarp and endosperm during corn nixtamalization—A review. Journal of Cereal Science. 2018;**81**:108-117

[93] Vázquez-Carrillo G, García-Cruz L, Molina-Macedo A, Marrufo-Diaz MDLL, Rodriguez-Garcia ME, Mier-Sainz Trapaga R, et al. Exploring the influence of wood ash, maize cob ash, and tequesquite (alkaline rock) on nixtamalization of maize. International Journal of Gastronomy and Food Science. 2024;**37**:100972

[94] Odjo S, Alakonya AE, Rosales-Nolasco A, Molina AL, Muñoz C, Palacios-Rojas N. Occurrence and postharvest strategies to help mitigate aflatoxins and fumonisins in maize and their co-exposure to consumers in Mexico and Central America. Food Control. 2022;**138**:108968

[95] Hamel R, Flowers K. Tracking promises analyzing the impact of feed the future in Guatemala [Internet]. Centre for Strategic and International Studies. 2019. Available from: https://gatesopenresearch.org/documents/3-1387

[96] De Campos M, Olszyna-Marzys AE. Aflatoxin contamination in grains and grain products during the dry season in Guatemala. Bulletin of Environmental Contamination and Toxicology. 1979;**22**:350-356

[97] De Campos M, Santos JC, Olszyna-Marzys AE. Aflatoxin contamination in grains from the Pacific coast in Guatemala and the effect of storage upon contamination. Bulletin of Environmental Contamination and Toxicology. 1980;**24**:789-795

[98] Mendoza R, Reen C, Stratton J, Hallen-adams HE. Understanding the Mycobiota of Maize from the Highlands of Guatemala, and Implications for Maize Quality and Safety. Vol. 101. Crop Protection. 2017. pp. 5-11

[99] Mendoza JR, Rodas A, Oliva A, Sabillón L, Colmenares A, Clarke J, et al. Safety and quality assessment of smallholder farmers' maize in the Western highlands of Guatemala. Journal of Food Protection. 2018;**81**:776-784

[100] Sabillón L, Alvarado J, Leiva A, Mendoza R, Espinal R, Leslie JF, et al. Presence, Co-occurrence, and daily intake estimates of aflatoxins and Fumonisins in maize consumed in food-insecure regions of Western Honduras. Toxins. 2023;**15**:559

[101] Julian AM, Wareing PW, Phillips SI, Medlock VFP, MacDonald MV, Del Río LE. Fungal contamination and selected mycotoxins in pre- and

post-harvest maize in Honduras. Mycopathologia. 1995;**129**:5-16

[102] Diaz GJ, Perilla NS, Rojas Y. Occurrence of aflatoxins in selected Columbian foods. Mycotoxin Research. 2001;**17**:15-20

[103] Mora M, Lacey J. Handling and aflatoxin contamination of white maize in Costa Rica. Mycopathologia. 1997;**138**:77-89

[104] Granados-Chinchilla F, Molina A, Chavarría G, Alfaro-Cascante M, Bogantes-Ledezma D, Murillo-Williams A. Aflatoxins occurrence through the food chain in Costa Rica: Applying the one health approach to mycotoxin surveillance. Food Control. 2017;**82**:217-226

[105] Martínez-Padrón HY, García-Olivares JG, MaG V-C, Mayek-Pérez N, Valdivia-Flores AG, Hernández-Delgado S. Physicochemical characteristics, mycoflora and aflatoxins in corn grown and stored in northern Tamaulipas, Mexico. Journal of Environmental Science and Health, Part B. 2024;**59**:737-747

[106] Molina-Pintor IB, Ruíz-Arias MA, Guerrero-Flores MC, Rojas-García AE, Barrón-Vivanco BS, Medina-Díaz IM, et al. Preliminary survey of the occurrence of mycotoxins in cereals and estimated exposure in a northwestern region of Mexico. International Journal of Environmental Health Research. 2022;**32**:2271-2285

[107] Aristil J. Aflatoxin contamination of baby food flour sold on Haitian markets. International Journal of Biological and Chemical Sciences. 2019;**13**:1821

[108] Sabino M, Prado G, Inomata EI, Pedroso MD, Garcia RV. Natural occurrence of aflatoxins and zearalenone in maize in Brazil. Part II. Food Additives & Contaminants. 1988;**6**:327-341

[109] Rocha LO, Nakai VK, Braghini R, Reis TA, Kobashigawa E, Corrêa B. Mycoflora and co-occurrence of fumonisins and aflatoxins in freshly harvested corn in different regions of Brazil. IJMS. 2009;**10**:5090-5103

[110] Oliveira CAF, Cruz JVS, Rosim RE, Bordin K, Kindermann ACP, Corassin CH. Simultaneous occurrence of aflatoxins and Fumonisins in corn intended for the pet feed industry and for human consumption. Journal of Food Chemistry and Nanotechnology. 2016;**2**(1). Available from: http://unitedscientificgroup.com/journals/ets/articles/v1n1/jfcn-004-oliveira-caf.html

[111] Bittencourt ABF, Oliveira CAF, Dilkin P, Corrêa B. Mycotoxin occurrence in corn meal and flour traded in São Paulo, Brazil. Food Control. 2005;**16**:117-120

[112] Amaral K, Nascimiento GB, Sekiyama BL, January V, Junior MM. Aflatoxins in corn-based products traded in Brazil and risks to human health. Food Science and Technology (Campinas). 2006;**26**:336-342

[113] Andrade PD, De Mello MH, França JA, Caldas ED. Aflatoxins in food products consumed in Brazil: A preliminary dietary risk assessment. Food Additives & Contaminants: Part A. 2013;**30**:127-136

[114] Noomhorn A, Cardona TD. Drying and chemical treatment of grains to prevent mycotoxin contamination during storage. In: Mycotoxin Prevention and Control in Food Grains. Food and Agriculture Organization of the United Nations

[115] Kaburi SA, Appiah F, Lamptey FP, Otoo GS. Controlling aflatoxin in maize:

The effects of varieties, packaging materials, and agroecological zones. Heliyon. 2023;**9**(11):e21645

[116] Purdue University. Purdue Improved Crop Storage Network Storing Safely to Stop Hunger [Internet]. 2015. Available from: https://picsnetwork.org/who-we-are/

[117] García-Lara S, García-Jaimes E, Ortíz-Islas S. Field effectiveness of improved hermetic storage technologies on maize grain quality in Central Mexico. Journal of Stored Products Research. 2020;**87**:101585

[118] Tubbs T, Baributsa D, Woloshuk C. Impact of opening hermetic storage bags on grain quality, fungal growth and aflatoxin accumulation. Journal of Stored Products Research. 2016;**69**:276-281

[119] Kiobia DO, Silayo VCK, Mutabazi KD, Graef F, Mourice SK. Performance of hermetic storage bags for maize grains under farmer-managed conditions: Good practice versus local reality. Journal of Stored Products Research. 2020;**87**:101586

[120] Hagler WM, Hutchins JE, Hamilton PB. Destruction of aflatoxin in corn with sodium bisulfite. Journal of Food Protection. 1982;**45**:1287-1291

[121] Moerck KE, Mcelfresh P, Wohlman A, Hilton BW. Aflatoxin destruction in corn using sodium bisulfite, sodium hydroxide and aqueous ammonia. Journal of Food Protection. 1980;**43**:571-574

[122] Stoloff L, Trucksess MW. Effect of boiling, frying, and baking on recovery of aflatoxin from naturally contaminated corn grits or cornmeal. Journal of the Association of Official Analytical Chemists. 1981;**64**:678-680

[123] Daba HG, Delele MA, Fanta SW, Habtu NG, Abera MK. Impact of traditional processing conditions and methods on the aflatoxin content of cooked maize. Cogent Food & Agriculture. 2024;**10**:2297516

[124] Odukoya JO, De Saeger S, De Boevre M, Adegoke GO, Devlieghere F, Croubels S, et al. Influence of traditional dehulling on mycotoxin reduction and GC-HRTOF-MS metabolites profile of fermented maize products. Heliyon. 2024;**10**:e23025

[125] Guzman-de-Pefia D, Trudel L, Wogan GN. Corn "Nixtamalizacion" and the fate of Radiolabelled aflatoxin B1 in the tortilla making process. Bulletin of Environmental Contamination and Toxicology. 1995;**55**:858-864

[126] Elias-Orozco R, Castellanos-Nava A, Gaytán-Martínez M, Figueroa-Cárdenas JD, Loarca-Piña G. Comparison of nixtamalization and extrusion processes for a reduction in aflatoxin content. Food Additives and Contaminants. 2002;**19**:878-885

[127] Méndez-Albores JA, Arámbula-Villa G, Loarca-Piña MG, González-Hernández J, Castaño-Tostado E, Moreno-Martínez E. Aflatoxins' fate during the nixtamalization of contaminated maize by two tortilla-making processes. Journal of Stored Products Research. 2004;**40**:87-94

[128] Montenegro-Benthancourt G, Glesener H, Torres O, Seegmiller E, Rohloff P, Voth-Gaeddert LE. Practices of maize handling and nixtamalization to reduce fungal toxin exposure in rural Guatemala. Journal of Agriculture and Food Research. 2024;**18**:101512

[129] Moreno-Pedraza A, Valdés-Santiago L, Hernández-Valadez LJ, Rodríguez-Sixtos Higuera A, Winkler R,

Guzmán-de Peña DL. Reduction of aflatoxin B1 during tortilla production and identification of degradation by-products by direct-injection electrospray mass spectrometry. Salud Publica de Mexico. 2015;**57**:50-57

[130] Torres P, Guzmán-Ortiz M, Ramírez-Wong B. Revising the role of pH and thermal treatments in aflatoxin content reduction during the tortilla and deep frying processes. Journal of Agricultural and Food Chemistry. 2001;**49**:2825-2829

[131] Cabrera-Meraz J, Maldonado L, Bianchini A, Espinal R. Incidence of aflatoxins and fumonisins in grain, masa and corn tortillas in four municipalities in the department of Lempira, Honduras. Heliyon. 2021;**7**:e08506

[132] Garsow AV, Torres OR, Matute JA, Voss DM, Miyagusuku-Cruzado G, Giusti MM, et al. Dietary, socioeconomic, and maize handling practices associated with aflatoxin and fumonisin exposure among women tortilla makers in 5 departments in Guatemala. PLOS Global Public Health. 2024;**4**:e0001623

[133] Twagiramungu JDD, Njoroge D, Mburu M, Duke G. Effect of Nixtamalization on aflatoxins, functional and acceptability of maize from Mulindi, Rwanda. EJFOOD. 2024;**6**:27-33

[134] Mannara C, Njue LG, Abong' GO. Dietary exposure of school children to aflatoxin and fumonisin through githeri and effectiveness of nixtamalization in reduction of these toxins in githeri from Turkana County. Mycotoxin Research. 2025;**41**:37-45

[135] Pérez-Flores GC, Moreno-Martínez E, Méndez-Albores A. Effect of microwave heating during alkaline-cooking of aflatoxin contaminated maize. Journal of Food Science. 2011;**76**:48-52

[136] Zavala-Franco A, Martinez-Flores HE, Vazquez-Duran AMAA. Fate of aflatoxins from a novel procedure for tortilla making based in infrared heating. The Philippine Agricultural Scientist. 2016;**99**:42-49

[137] Zavala-Franco A, Canelo-Álvarez F, García-Salinas F, Alcántara-Zavala A, Figueroa-Cárdenas JDD, Méndez-Albores A. Evaluation of the nixtamalized cornbread-making process as a method of aflatoxin detoxification. Journal of Consumer Protection and Food Safety. 2024;**19**(1):71-80

[138] Bullerman LB, Bianchini A. Stability of mycotoxins during food processing. International Journal of Food Microbiology. 2007;**119**(1-2):140-146

[139] Sohi Sukham K, Sharma NS, Bobade H, Singh B, Sharma S. Effect of extrusion variables (moisture content, barrel temperature and screw speed) on the reduction of aflatoxins in maize. International Research Journal of Biological Sciences. 2015;**4**:31-37

[140] Massarolo KC, Mendoza JR, Verma T, Kupski L, Badiale-Furlong E, Bianchini A. Fate of aflatoxins in cornmeal during single-screw extrusion: A bioaccessibility approach. Lwt. 2021;**138**(2020)

[141] Castillo-Urueta P, Carvajal M, Méndez I, Meza F, Gálvez A. Survey of aflatoxins in maize tortillas from Mexico City. Food Additives & Contaminants: Part B. 2011;**4**(1):42-51

[142] Kroker-Lobos MF, Alvarez CS, Rivera-Andrade A, Smith JW, Egner P, Torres O, et al. Association between aflatoxin-albumin adduct levels and tortilla consumption in

Guatemalan adults. Toxicology Reports. 2019;**6**:465-471

[143] Sandoval IG, Wesseling S, Tietjens MCM. Aflatoxin B1 in nixtamalized maize in Mexico; occurrence and accompanying risk assessment. Toxicology Reports. 2019;**6**:1135-1142

[144] Zuki-Orozco BA, Batres-Esquivel LE, Ortiz-Pérez MD, Juárez-Flores BI, Díaz-Barriga F. Aflatoxins contamination in maize products from rural communities in San Luis Potosi, Mexico. Annals of Global Health. 2018;**84**(2):300-305

[145] Calvert L, Izquierdo J. Rice Production in Latin America at Critical Crossroads. (International Rice Commission Newsletter). Report No.: 55; 2006 p. 65-73

[146] Sanint LR. Rice-based production systems for food security and poverty alleviation in Latin America and the Caribbean. In: Proceedings of the FAO Rice Conference Rice Is Life [Internet]. Food and Agriculture Organization of the United Nations: Rome, Italy; 2004. Available from: https://www.fao.org/4/y5682e/y5682e0e.htm#TopOfPage

[147] Zorrilla G, Martínez C, Berrío L, Corredor E, Carmona L, Pulver E. Improving Rice production Systems in Latin America and the Caribbean. In: Eco Efficiency from Vision to Reality. 2012

[148] Chaudhari PR, Tamrakar N, Singh L, Tandon A, Sharma D. Rice nutritional and medicinal properties: A review article. Journal of Pharmacognosy and Phytochemistry. 2018;7:150-156

[149] Kalita T, Hazarika J. Morphological study, nutritional value and phytochemical estimation of four indigenous rice (*Oryza sativa* L.) varieties of Assam, India. Food Research. 2022;**6**(1):196-203

[150] Ahmed F, Mia S, Thongrak S, Kiatpathomchai S. Production, postharvest technology and trade of rice: A study on the current scenario in Asean. International Journal of Management. 2020;**11**:1373-1384

[151] Fukagawa NK, Ziska LH. Rice: Importance for global nutrition. Journal of Nutritional Science and Vitaminology. 2019;**65**(Supplement):S2-S3

[152] U.S. Food and Drug Administration. Arsenic in Rice and Rice Products Risk Assessment Report [Internet]. 2016. Available from: https://www.fda.gov/files/food/published/Arsenic-in-Rice-and-Rice-Products-Risk-Assessment-Report-PDF

[153] Boers HM, Seijen Ten Hoorn J, Mela DJ. A systematic review of the influence of rice characteristics and processing methods on postprandial glycaemic and insulinaemic responses. The British Journal of Nutrition. 2015;**114**:1035-1045

[154] Naeem I, Ismail A, Riaz M, Aziz M, Akram K, Shahzad MA, et al. Aflatoxins in the rice production chain: A review on prevalence, detection, and decontamination strategies. Food Research International. 2024;**188**:114441

[155] Katsurayama AM, Martins LM, Iamanaka BT, Fungaro MHP, Silva JJ, Frisvad JC, et al. Occurrence of aspergillus section Flavi and aflatoxins in Brazilian rice: From field to market. International Journal of Food Microbiology. 2018;**266**:213-221

[156] Trucksess MW, Abbas HK, Weaver CM, Shier WT. Distribution of aflatoxins in shelling and milling fractions of naturally contaminated rice.

Food Additives & Contaminants: Part A. 2011;**28**:1076-1082

[157] Gunasekara DS. A brief review: Occurrence of aflatoxins in raw and parboiled rice in Sri Lankan market. AFSJ. 2022;**21**:119-124

[158] Dors GC, de Almeida A, Pinto L, Badiale-Furlong E. Migration of mycotoxins into rice starchy endosperm during the parboiling process. LWT - Food Science and Technology. 2009;**42**(1):433-437

[159] Bandara JMRS, Vithanege AK, Bean GA. Occurrence of aflatoxins in parboiled rice in Sri Lanka. Mycopathologia. 1991 Nov;**116**(2):65-70

[160] Iqbal SZ, Asi MR, Ariño A, Akram N, Zuber M. Aflatoxin contamination in different fractions of rice from Pakistan and estimation of dietary intakes. Mycotoxin Research. 2012;**28**(3):175-180

[161] Corrêa ANR, Ferreira CD. Mycotoxins in grains and cereals intended for human consumption: Brazilian legislation, occurrence above maximum levels and co-occurrence. Food Reviews International. 2023;**39**:5920-5933

[162] Barbosa NA, Fernandes AM, De Oliveira SL, De Castro F, Burbarelli M, Lopes De Oliveira A, et al. Occurrence of aflatoxins in organic rice produced and commercialized in Brazil. Food Control. 2024;**166**:110764

[163] Sani AM, Azizi EG, Salehi EA, Rahimi K. Reduction of aflatoxin in rice by different cooking methods. Toxicology and Industrial Health. 2014;**30**:546-550

[164] Romero-Sánchez I, Gracia-Lor E, Madrid-Albarrán Y. Aflatoxin detoxification by thermal cooking treatment and evaluation of in vitro bioaccessibility from white and brown rice. Food Chemistry. 2024;**436**:137738

[165] Park J, Kim Y. Effect of pressure cooking on aflatoxin B1 in Rice. Journal of Agricultural and Food Chemistry. 2006;**54**:2431-2435

[166] da Silva MN, Massarolo KC, Kupski L, Furlong EB. Hydrothermal treatment of rice: Reduction of aflatoxins and bioaccessibility. Journal of Cereal Science. 2019;**85**:199-205